WHAT STATE DO YOU LIVE IN?

The Consequences of Obesity

REVISED EDITION

Six Levels of Proven Food Strategies to
Reverse and Manage Insulin Resistance

JERROD P. LIBONATI, MS, RD

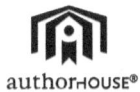
authorHOUSE®

AuthorHouse™
1663 Liberty Drive
Bloomington, IN 47403
www.authorhouse.com
Phone: 1-800-839-8640

© 2011 Jerrod P. Libonati, MS, RD. All rights reserved.

No part of this book may be reproduced, stored in a retrieval system, or transmitted by any means without the written permission of the author.

First published by AuthorHouse 4/04/2011

ISBN: 978-1-4567-4093-1 (sc)
ISBN: 978-1-4567-4105-1 (dj)
ISBN: 978-1-4567-4094-8 (e)

Library of Congress Control Number: 2011902694

Printed in the United States of America

Any people depicted in stock imagery provided by Thinkstock are models, and such images are being used for illustrative purposes only.
Certain stock imagery © Thinkstock.

This book is printed on acid-free paper.

Because of the dynamic nature of the Internet, any web addresses or links contained in this book may have changed since publication and may no longer be valid. The views expressed in this work are solely those of the author and do not necessarily reflect the views of the publisher, and the publisher hereby disclaims any responsibility for them.

Contents

Section I	**The Healthy State**	1
Chapter 1	Carbohydrates	3
Chapter 2	Excess Glucose Equals Body Fat	5
Chapter 3	Fat in The Food You Eat	6
Chapter 4	Dietary Cholesterol	10
Chapter 5	Fat Cells	13
Chapter 6	Insulin & The Disposal Business	15
Chapter 7	Fat & Cholesterol Metabolism	19
Chapter 8	Fat Floating Compounds	21
Chapter 9	Insulin Controls Carbohydrate & Fat Metabolism	23
Chapter 10	HDL Cholesterol	25
Chapter 11	The Birth of LDL Cholesterol	27
Chapter 12	HDL's & LDL's	29
Chapter 13	Energy Regulation	32
Section II	**The Insulin Resistant State**	35
Chapter 14	Abnormal Blood Glucose	37
Chapter 15	Fat Compartments	40
Chapter 16	Insulin Resistance & High Blood Fats	43
Chapter 17	Insulin Resistance & Lower HDL Cholesterol	46
Chapter 18	Insulin Resistance & Your Muscles	48
Chapter 19	Your Toxic Blood	50
Chapter 20	High Blood Pressure	52

Chapter 21	The Metabolic Syndrome	57
Chapter 22	Heart Disease	61

Section III	**The Great Diet Debate**	**63**
Chapter 23	Reversing Weight Related Insulin Resistance	65
Chapter 24	Lower Fat Diets & Insulin Resistance	67
Chapter 25	Lower Carb Diets & Insulin Resistance	75
Chapter 26	Supplements & Insulin Resistance	79

Section IV	**The Food Strategies**	**83**
Chapter 27	Weight Related Insulin Resistant Food Strategies	85

Abbreviations

CARBS	Carbohydrates
CVD	Cardiovascular disease
FFC	Fat floating compound
HDL	High density lipoprotein
HSL	Hormone Sensitive Lipase
LDL	Low density lipoprotein
LPL	Lipoprotein lipase
MUFA	Monounsaturated fat
PUFA	Polyunsaturated fat
SAT FAT	Saturated fat
VLDL	Very low density lipoprotein

Introduction

Weight gain through adulthood, we all experience it, attempt to do something about it, and sadly, accept it. Most adults feel it's really nothing to worry about. After all, you feel fine and the only drawbacks are not being able to tuck your shirt in, having to buy larger pants, and breathing a bit harder as you walk up the stairs. Unfortunately, the events linked to long term weight gain promote insulin resistance.

Insulin resistance is a condition where insulin is unable to properly dispose of dietary carbohydrate. The early stages of insulin resistance appear as "slightly high blood sugar". It's actually pre-diabetes and your chance to stop the progression of type two (type II) diabetes. Don't ignore this state. Glucose (blood sugar), fat, cholesterol, and insulin are destroying your arteries, liver, and pancreas. Immediate action is required to reverse what years of faulty nutrition and a lack of motivation has promoted.

What State Do You Live in The Consequences of Obesity begins with you in the healthy state. It describes normal carbohydrate, fat, and cholesterol metabolism. The story progresses into the insulin resistant state detailing "how" and "why" excess body weight promotes insulin resistance. Understanding both states, healthy and unhealthy, will help motivate you to begin taking the necessary steps to reverse what's not visible. Knowledge is power and you simply cannot know enough about the progression of weight related insulin resistance, a disease that promotes many forms of heart disease including high blood pressure, abnormal blood cholesterol and triglycerides, and type II diabetes.

There are several essential ingredients of the story you should be aware of. First, the story does not promote any unrealistic approach to treating and managing weight related insulin resistance. There are no promises or "magic" bullets at the end of the story. In fact, the story promotes food, not pills, supplements, or any other form of synthetic nutrition to treat a weight-food related condition. This book offers flexibility and allows you to choose the level and type of food strategy that establishes motivating habits. It discusses the pros and cons of current food prescriptions such as lower fat versus lower carbohydrate for reversing weight related insulin resistance. Six levels of food strategies, some as simple as snacking are included to put you on the right track in making realistic and necessary lifestyle changes to prevent a heart attack or stroke.

If you are looking to understand the progression of weight related diseased states and how to reverse them, read this story. If you are looking for food strategies that educate and teach you how to effectively manage your nutrition, this book is for you. Don't ignore the overweight or pre-obese state as I like to call it. It's likely the root of many cardiovascular disease (CVD) states. Prevention through nutrition, not medication, is your only true means of protection against diet and weight related disease.

SECTION I
THE HEALTHY STATE

1 CARBOHYDRATES

Carbohydrates (carbs) are in nearly everything you consume. Fruit, fruit juice, dried fruit, and *all* vegetables are 100% carbs, which many don't realize. Grain products such as cereal, bread, oatmeal, rice, pastas, waffles, and pancakes are also examples of carbs. Starchy foods such as potatoes, sweet potatoes, yams, corn, and peas are classified as carbs, as are beans and legumes, even though they do provide protein. Snack foods and desserts such as chips, cookies, cakes, pies, ice creams, frozen yogurts, and candy are rich in carbs. Beverages including soda, beer, wine, liquor, and energy drinks are also classified as carbs. As you can see, carbs are everywhere. The easiest way to determine if a food or beverage contains carbohydrate is to look at the nutrition facts panel. If the panel lists total carbohydrates, then you can be assured the product contains sugar, the end result of digested carbohydrate.

All Roads Lead to Glucose

Carbohydrate metabolism begins as soon as the carbohydrate portion of the food or drink enters your mouth. To use carbohydrates, your body must have it available in the most efficient and profitable form of sugar called glucose. As glucose enters the blood, levels begin to rise. This newly elevated blood glucose is temporary and normal. As your cells use the glucose, blood levels return to normal. All cells use glucose in one way or another, but the focus will be on your liver, muscle, and fat cells.

Glucose in Your Liver

Your liver is the main site of glucose metabolism. It satisfies two immediate requirements when glucose enters. Some glucose is "burned" for energy like your vehicle burns gasoline and some glucose is stored, not as fat, but as glucose reserves. The fancy name for liver glucose is glycogen. Your liver holds about one third of your total body glycogen. Your liver, when it needs to, breaks glycogen down and converts it back to glucose. Additionally, your liver is so sophisticated it has the ability to produce glucose from protein rich sources such as meat and poultry.

Glucose in Your Muscles

Much of the glucose traveling in the blood is taken up and used by your muscle cells. Muscles act very similar to your liver in the way they handle glucose. Muscles burn glucose for energy and store glucose as glycogen. In fact, muscles store two thirds of your total body glycogen.

Muscles engaged in daily (regular) exercise help regulate blood glucose. It may be used as energy or stored as glycogen. However your muscles decide to use glucose, the bottom line is they help lower and maintain healthy blood glucose levels.

Glucose for Your Brain, Pancreas, and Kidneys

Some blood glucose travels to your pancreas, kidneys, and brain to be used as fuel. In fact, your brain thrives on glucose. While it can run on fats, it prefers glucose. Fueling your brain with fats or with very little carbohydrate is like adding water to your gas tank. Your vehicle will run very inefficiently and not for long before problems develop. All three cellular communities along with your liver and muscles help maintain normal blood glucose.

2 Excess Glucose Equals Body Fat

If glucose entering your liver is determined to be excess, meaning other cells have received their glucose fix, it becomes fat. Excess glucose will be converted into triglycerides, the universal storage form of fat in the body. In the liver, triglycerides may interfere with glucose processing. To ensure that fat and glucose metabolism remain separate, triglycerides are placed in a temporary holding tank known as a triglyceride pool. What happens with these triglycerides will alarm you. This is explained in great detail in section two, the insulin resistant state.

Excess Glucose in Your Blood

If glucose continues entering your liver, it will be released back into the blood. To prevent glucose accumulation in the blood, your stomach fat cells act as perfect fat holding tanks. Once excess glucose enters stomach fat cells, it is converted into a triglyceride and stored, exactly the same way your liver handles triglycerides. Years of excess glucose, resulting from carbohydrate overeating can be stored as triglycerides in your stomach fat cells. Unfortunately, as we age, fat becomes visually noticeable and unappealing as fat cells become overly packed with triglycerides.

3 Fat in The Food You Eat

Fat in the food you eat is called dietary fat. Dietary fat exists in nearly every food. Believe it or not, fruit and vegetables such as apples, bananas, and broccoli contain traces of fat. Even if a food label lists "0" grams of total fat, the food may not be truly fat free. Labeling laws allow manufacturers to list zero next to total fat grams if the serving size contains less than a half gram of total fat per serving. Of course you should continue eating fruit and vegetables. They are full of water, fiber, vitamins, and minerals that are integral to reversing and managing your weight related insulin resistant state.

Do You Need Fat in Your Diet?

You need dietary fat to live. While fats provide energy (calories) and structure for every cell in your body, they also accomplish the task of regulating hormones. Insulin, a hormone you're going to learn all about, is partially controlled by stored fats. In the absence of glucose, fats are released from fat cells (storage depots) where they travel to and stimulate the pancreas to produce and secrete insulin. Of course you don't want your fat cells to release too much fat into the blood, so this action of liberating stored fat is a tightly controlled process.

Types of Fat

There are four types of dietary fat. Fat exists as monounsaturated (mufa), polyunsaturated (pufa), saturated (sat fat), and trans-fat. Under total fat grams listed on a food label, there is usually a breakdown of the individual types of fat that exist within the total fat. If you add up the individual grams of each fat type, their sum must equal the total fat grams listed. For example, if the label lists 8 grams of total fat, two grams may come from mufa, four grams from pufa, and the remainder from either saturated or trans-fat or both. In general, it is best to consume mufas and pufas as saturated and trans-fat are clearly linked to heart and artery disease. In fact, it would be safe to eliminate saturated and trans-fat altogether as mufas and pufas are able to serve all necessary purposes.

Take the avocado for example. It's a fruit that's well recognized for its contribution of "good" fats, the mufas and pufas. This is the "preferred fat profile" that you should look for when reading food labels. Many vegetable oils have a large percentage of total fat in the form of mufa and pufa. The two with the highest are olive oil and canola oil. Nuts are also a good source while being relatively low in saturated fat. Of course you will have to exercise portion control as fat, regardless of the type or source is rich in calories. Ultimately, your stomach fat cells don't discriminate against "good" or "bad" fats (calories). Any type of calorie in excess will be converted into and stored as body fat in the form of triglycerides.

Dietary Triglycerides

When you consume dietary fat, you're really eating a composite of mufa, pufa, sat fat, and trans-fat. You're not just consuming a single type of fat. Most often, you're consuming at least two or three types of dietary fat in a single food. Dietary fat exists as triglycerides, which are three individual fats linked together forming a single larger fat. For example, when you eat avocado, no matter if you slice it into a salad or make it into a spread, you're eating mufas, pufas, and a bit of sat fat linked together to form a triglyceride. Dietary triglycerides can be composed of three identical fats such as three pufas or three mufas or any combination of the four types of fat. If you look at the fat grams on food labels you should be concerned with two pieces of information. First, make sure the product is low in total fat per serving. Second and this is the most critical part of choosing the product, make sure the majority of fats come from mufa and pufa, and not saturated or trans fat. All foods provided for you in the food strategies section have this profile.

The Best Fat, Mufa vs. Pufa

I am sure that you are wondering about the "best" type of fat. Since you already know mufas and pufas are preferred over sat fat, then of the two, which is best? Since both help lower LDL cholesterol, I rank them equal in terms of "best". Your snack and food strategies are full of these unsaturated "heart healthy" fats!

Pufa vs. Pufa

Polyunsaturated fat exist in two forms, omega 6's and omega 3's. Both are essential and must come from foods you eat. Omega 6 fats are the predominant type of pufa fat in the American diet. Vegetable oils such as corn, sunflower, safflower, canola, olive, and soybean oil used in cooking and to produce many baked goods are the main sources.

Omega 3's on the other hand, are not so widespread. They are found primarily in coldwater fish and a few plants. Fish sources include salmon, trout, and certain tunas. Plant sources include walnuts and flaxseeds. Unfortunately, fish sources are often left out of the daily diet as taste and convenience outweighs the benefits.

Here's the deal. While omega 6's are "good" fats as they help lower your "bad" cholesterol, they are over consumed compared to omega 3's. Typically, most adults consume more than 20 times the amount of omega 6's compared to omega 3's. Unfortunately, this skewed ratio isn't the best situation for treating weight related insulin resistance. All complete food strategies in section four provide balanced ratios of omega 6 and omega 3 pufas.

Saturated Fat

Saturated fats will raise your "bad" or low-density lipoprotein (LDL) cholesterol. Although saturated fat may raise your "good" or high-density lipoprotein (HDL) cholesterol, it's not worth the risk as it will likely lead to a greater increase in LDL cholesterol. In section two, I will provide you with the "best" non-pharmacological way to improve HDL cholesterol.

Trans-fat

Trans-fat is twice as bad as sat fat. They raise your LDL cholesterol and lower your HDL cholesterol. Stay clear of trans-fat which is found in foods of animal origin such as red meat, full fat dairy products, and plant oils that contain partially hydrogenated vegetable oil.

4 Dietary Cholesterol

Animal foods such as milk, cheese, eggs, beef, chicken, pork, and fish contain cholesterol known as dietary cholesterol. Plant foods on the other hand, such as fruit, vegetables, whole grains like brown rice and oatmeal, nuts and seeds, and legumes, contain fat, but never have and never will contain cholesterol. Only food of animal origin contains dietary cholesterol. For example, the avocado we discussed earlier does contain fat, but it does not contain any dietary cholesterol since it's a fruit.

Cholesterol Production

Cholesterol is so vital to your health that nearly every cell in your body comes equipped with machinery to produce it. Each day, you liver, the largest producer of cholesterol, manufactures approximately 1,000 milligrams (mg). To give you an idea of how much that is, an average size egg contains 70-75 milligrams of dietary cholesterol.

Cholesterol is made in your liver by metabolizing carbohydrate, protein, and fat. During this process, "fragments" from these nutrients are assembled into cholesterol globules. Over eating any one of these nutrients prompts your liver to produce even more cholesterol. Millions of adults suffer from the overproduction of hepatic (liver) cholesterol, which contributes to high blood cholesterol and increases your risk of heart and artery disease significantly. While nearly all cells produce cholesterol, only your liver's production of cholesterol has the ability to raise your blood cholesterol.

Why Is Cholesterol So Important?

Cholesterol acts as a "spacer" for cells. Here's a clearer picture. Inside the tires of your vehicle, there are steel belts. The steel belts, while holding tire components together, act as a spacer between the layers of rubber. This is exactly how cholesterol works in your cells. It lodges itself between rows of fat that make up the outer lining of your cells. The "spacing" of cholesterol between fats prevents your cells from becoming stiff and impermeable. This allows for effective cell stimulation and efficient nutrient and fluid exchange. Chronic disease states progress when cells lose their ability to communicate and exchange nutrients and fluids.

Cholesterol is also used to make several important hormones such as estrogen, testosterone, Vitamin D, and the emulsifying compound bile. Bile is an emulsifier, a compound that mixes dietary fat and cholesterol together, thereby increasing their absorption efficiency.

Stop Eating Foods with Cholesterol

You should stop consuming dietary cholesterol for several reasons. First, your liver produces all of the cholesterol you need each day. If you consume dietary cholesterol, your liver recognizes this and in turn decreases its own production to regulate the amount that ends up in the blood. This is not saying blood cholesterol isn't influenced by dietary cholesterol, it is, but it doesn't raise your blood cholesterol too significantly.

Controlling Cholesterol Production

There is a simple way to lower your total blood cholesterol. Eat smaller meals. Spreading your calories throughout the day versus eating one or two large meals keeps cholesterol production under control. Eating too many calories all at once not only makes you feel tired and lethargic, but the masses of insulin released from your pancreas in response to the carbohydrate portion of the meal or snack, speeds up the production of cholesterol in your liver! Spreading calories evenly across the day helps you in three ways. First, it begins teaching you portion control. Second, it shrinks your stomach. Third, it prevents excess cholesterol production. It's a win win situation for you! In all food strategies, calories and carbohydrates have been spaced evenly throughout the day to prevent unwanted cholesterol production.

Fiber Lowers Total Cholesterol

Of the many notable features of fiber including cancer prevention, diabetes management, and gastrointestinal (GI) health, one stands out when it comes to lowering your risk of heart disease. As fiber is metabolized, it binds to bile, a compound that aids in dietary fat and cholesterol metabolism. Once bound to bile, fiber is excreted. Bile that is lost by fiber elimination must be replaced. To compensate for the loss of bile, blood cholesterol is taken up by your liver and used to produce new bile. This process lowers your blood cholesterol. Therefore, each and every time you consume fibrous foods, you are lowering your total blood cholesterol. Each snack and meal strategy provides you with ample dietary fiber, a necessary tool in the fight against abnormal blood cholesterol and heart and artery disease.

5 Fat Cells

You have fat cells everywhere, in all areas of your body. Unfortunately, this means you can become fat just about anywhere. Fat cells are quite unique. They protect you from common chronic disease states such as weight related insulin resistance, atherosclerosis, and type two diabetes. Fat cells, and let's focus on your stomach fat cells, perform two main jobs.

Stomach Fat Cells

Their first job and quite possibly their most important is to store excess calories. Nutrients such as glucose and protein that are consumed above your needs will be converted into and stored as triglycerides. The storage of dietary fat is less complicated. It doesn't require any processing before being stored as a triglyceride. It's simply escorted into fat cells, linked with other individual fats into a triglyceride and stored. Although body fat is unappealing and unhealthy, as long as fat cells continue to store triglycerides, they're actually protecting you and your blood. If excess glucose, protein, and fat (calories) were to remain circulating across your arteries, heart disease would appear at a very young age. Once a triglyceride is formed, it's neatly packed away in your fat cells. Fat cells store decades worth of triglycerides, a preventive process as fats and glucose left circulating in the blood would become toxic. You will find out just how dirty and polluted your blood is likely to become if your body weight begins to promote insulin resistance.

Their second job is to release stored fat. In times of low blood glucose (energy), fat cells act as "energy releasing warehouses" by releasing fat into the blood. For example, your heart cells constantly require fuel. At night, when glucose may not be available, fats are released into the blood where they travel to and feed your heart to keep it beating. Fat cells are simply giant fat warehouses. They are stimulated to take fuel out of your blood only to release the fuel back into your blood when needed. Many chronic "dieters" believe that fat cells have a preference and only store excess carbohydrate calories as fat. This is not true.

Fat Cell Growth

Your stomach fat cells are not like balloons. They don't continue expanding if you fill them with excess calories (triglycerides). Stomach fat cells have a "fat capacity". They can only be stuffed to a certain size before they divide into two new smaller fat cells. As long as you continue taking in excess calories, *your fat cells will keep growing to a certain size and dividing*. You can become infinitely fat as each new fat cell comes equipped with fat making and storing capabilities. There is one big problem with gaining body fat, fat cells never go away. In other words, when you lose weight, you don't lose fat cells. They only shrink and their propensity to re-inflate is dependent on your intake of calories.

6 Insulin & The Disposal Business

Immediately following a carbohydrate meal or snack, blood glucose levels begin to rise. Your pancreas instantly recognizes this elevation and begins producing and shipping insulin into the blood. Much of the initial shipment of insulin into the blood heads for your liver where it begins multi tasking. Other shipments of insulin are sent to all parts of your body where the blood glucose lowering "process" begins.

Lowering Blood Glucose

Insulin has several roles when it comes to controlling and maintaining "healthy and acceptable" blood glucose levels. First, the most noted role of insulin is to help lower elevated blood glucose. Blood glucose is lowered as insulin demands your cells to open up and take in glucose. As glucose leaves the blood and enters your cells, blood glucose levels begin returning to their healthy and normal range. Each and every time you consume carbohydrate food or beverage, this process takes place to ensure "healthy and acceptable" blood glucose levels.

When is Insulin Produced?

The instant carbohydrate digestion takes place, which begins on your tongue, your pancreas begins producing insulin. Sounds strange, but your pancreas has "glucose sensors" that recognize even the slightest increase in blood glucose. The more carbohydrate you consume, the higher your blood glucose and blood insulin levels. It's a one to one ratio. This creates two conditions, hyperglycemia and hyperinsulinemia. Both states are temporary and normal following carbohydrate consumption. Within a few hours, blood glucose and insulin concentrations diminish and return to their "normal and acceptable" ranges.

Insulin and Glucose Disposal

It's hard to imagine, but insulin arrives at your cells ahead of glucose. Let's take a look at how insulin works when it arrives at your muscle cells. The arrival of insulin at your muscles resembles the space shuttle arriving at the space station to begin a mission. The space shuttle must dock to the space station in a very precise manner. If it fails to line up perfectly or if the docking station is obstructed or dysfunctional, the space shuttle cannot land and the mission will be aborted. Insulin works the same way. If insulin is not allowed to dock to the insulin receptor on the cell, glucose levels will remain higher than normal for a greater length of time.

Insulin and Your Muscles

Your muscles are giant glucose furnaces and warehouses only if the glucose is inside your muscles. How does it get inside?

The docking of insulin to the insulin receptor sends a "signal" to the center of your muscle cell. This signal informs the entire muscle cell that glucose has arrived and is waiting to enter. The signal not only informs the muscle cell that it needs to open, it activates glucose transporters. As glucose begins flowing into your muscles, transporters within the cell help direct glucose towards usage or storage. This entire process lowers your temporary state of hyperglycemia.

Insulin and Your Fat Cells

The docking of and stimulating process by insulin on fat cells is identical to that of muscle cells. The difference is your pancreas and arteries take a direct hit. As your weight escalates which increases the number of fat cells, greater demand is placed on your pancreas. More insulin is required to stimulate the increased number of fat cells. While this process does lower your blood glucose, the temporary state of hyperinsulinemia begins damaging your arteries and promoting high blood pressure. While insulin is busy stimulating your muscles and fat cells to properly dispose of glucose, it's performing other important duties as well.

Inhibitory Feature One

As insulin is in the process of regulating blood glucose, it simultaneously inhibits your liver from releasing glucose into the blood. Here's why. If glucose is present following a meal or snack, there's no need to increase levels as this would lead to even higher blood sugar. To prevent this undesirable event, insulin is able to trump your liver and suppress glucose release.

Inhibitory Feature Two

As insulin is suppressing liver glucose release, it's inhibiting the release of stored triglycerides from fat cells. Let me explain this one. If you have glucose circulating in your blood, there's no need for any other type of fuel, from either glucose or fat. To ensure that no other fuels leak into your blood, insulin is powerful enough to inhibit the release of stored triglycerides from stomach fat cells.

Why Insulin Needs to Be Powerful

Imagine how your blood looks after you finish a snack or meal containing carbohydrate and fat? There is glucose and fat circulating through your blood waiting to be directed into their appropriate places. Now imagine insulin loses its controlling and influential powers. What if it fails to inhibit glucose release from your liver? What if triglycerides begin seeping from fat cells? Where would all of this glucose and fat end up?

Other All Important Features of Insulin

Insulin helps promote normal blood pressure. In the normal and healthy state insulin helps with blood flow and therefore the circulation and distribution of nutrients by keeping blood vessels open. This action, called vasodilation, prevents high blood pressure.

Insulin also plays a key role in appetite reduction. In the brain, it acts as a "satiety signal", triggering fullness and therefore cessation of eating!

Insulin Summary

Insulin is essential to your cells and serves many important roles. Primarily, insulin protects your blood from becoming a toxic river of glucose by stimulating muscle and fat cells to lower blood glucose. Protective roles of insulin include;
- Preventing your liver from releasing glucose
- Protecting you from sustained hyperglycemia
- Inhibiting the release of stored fats into the blood
- Promoting normal blood pressure
- Acting as a satiety signal

7 Fat & Cholesterol Metabolism

Chewing your food is the initial step in digesting dietary fat. In your mouth, dietary fat is attacked by enzymes capable of breaking down dietary triglycerides into smaller fats. In your stomach, fats are separated according to how long they are. Sounds odd, but the length or size of the fat determines its fate. If dietary cholesterol is present, it is separated from the fat. Left floating are individual dietary fats and cholesterol if present as both do not mix with the watery environment of your stomach.

Absorption of Small and Medium Fats

Smaller and medium length fats are soluble enough to leave your intestine unassisted. They are used by your liver and muscles for energy, just like glucose. Insulin stimulation is not required for uptake and use of these fats. Don't rush out and begin researching what foods contain only small and medium length fats as a way to prevent fat storage. This won't work. Most food contains a mixture of dietary small, medium, and long length fats.

Absorption of Longer Length Fats

Longer length fats are too big to be absorbed into the blood. They require assistance prior to being transported through the blood. Long length fats are combined back into triglycerides in your intestinal cells. Cholesterol, if present may be incorporated into these triglycerides. You start off eating fat in the form of a dietary triglyceride only to be broken down and reformed back into a triglyceride.

Reforming a triglyceride in the intestine doesn't help with the solubility of the triglycerides. To help solve this problem, triglycerides are assigned a guide. This guide is a protein, but not the type that comes from eating chicken or fish. Rather, this protein is produced in response to the insolubility of dietary fat and cholesterol. Masses of triglycerides are grouped together while the guide attaches itself. The fancy name of these large triglyceride compounds is chylomicron, but to keep things simple, they will be referred to as fat floating compounds or FFC's for the remainder of the story.

8 Fat Floating Compounds

The FFC's are ready to be released into the blood, but they're not. If all FFC's were released into the blood at once, your blood would become full of fat and cholesterol, giving it a murky appearance. Remember walking through water with mud on your shoes as a kid? As the mud dissolved, the water became very cloudy. To prevent this, FFC's are transported through a series of alternate channels that run parallel to your blood vessels. These channels are your lymphatic vessels. Just prior to the lymphatic vessels emptying into the blood, FFC's are halted by a gatekeeper. His job is to prevent the massive release of FFC's into the blood. Only a small amount of FFC's are allowed into the blood every few minutes.

The Attack on FFC's
Unfortunately, FFC's are released into the blood right near your heart. This means, your arteries that lie on top of your heart, your coronary arteries, are one of the first groups of blood vessels to receive this initial shipment of FFC's. Over time, fats and cholesterol are likely to accumulate in these arteries, promoting the progression of heart and artery disease.

FFC's are attacked as they travel in the blood. Lying on the surface of stomach fat cells, and all fat cells for that matter is LPL, a triglyceride thief. LPL is born on your fat cells, lives on the outside of your fat cells, and spends much of your adult life stealing triglycerides from FFC's as they pass through your arteries. LPL is able to travel and relocate to other cellular communities like your muscle cells, but prefers your fat cells, where fat should be stored. If LPL relocates and begins escorting fats into muscles, you're in big trouble as muscles are giant glucose furnaces and warehouses. As you are well aware, there seems to be endless storage room in fat cells as evidenced by a progressive widening of the American waist line.

What Happens During the Attack?

The guide that was initially attached to FFC's that offered guidance and solubility caused the attack on purpose. Without the guide, LPL would have no way to "sense" triglycerides within FFC's. LPL steals mainly triglycerides from FFC's. As much as 80% of the triglycerides are stolen. Triglycerides are broken down into individual fats, escorted into your stomach fat cells, and reassembled back into triglycerides, the universal storage form of fat in your body.

Inside Your Fat Cells

Inside your fat cells, triglycerides are protected by HSL, a triglyceride watch guard. HSL's role is to prevent triglycerides from escaping back into the blood. When LPL is stealing triglycerides, HSL is inactive as it functions to safeguard triglycerides.

After the Attack

Following the attacks on FFC's, a few triglycerides, as most were stolen, and the majority of dietary cholesterol (if present in the food you ate) remain circulating in your blood. While your liver is busy processing and storing glucose, it now has to deal with some triglycerides and a whole bunch of cholesterol that begins entering. Keep in mind this process is continuous. FFC's are entering the blood every few minutes for over 10 hours after you eat a meal containing dietary fat and cholesterol.

Dietary fat and cholesterol metabolism is now complete. Smaller and medium length fats are burned as energy just like carbohydrates, while longer length fats end up being stored in your fat cells as triglycerides or being removed from the blood by your liver along with cholesterol if present, following LPL attacks.

9 Insulin Controls Carbohydrate & Fat Metabolism

In the normal state, insulin simultaneously controls glucose and fat metabolism.

If insulin is present in the blood, it indicates one of two situations. First, it signals to your entire body that glucose is present and no other type of fuel is necessary to provide your cells with energy. If this is the case, HSL, the triglyceride watch guard, is inactivated by insulin's presence. This prevents fats from leaving fat cells. Second, when insulin is present, it has the ability to regulate LPL. As insulin is busy stimulating cells to dispose of glucose, it stimulates LPL, the triglyceride thief just in case dietary fat and cholesterol (in FFC's) may be entering the blood. In other words, insulin is a multi-tasking hormone that prepares your cells for nutrient metabolism.

When Does HSL Become Active?

When you're resting or sleeping or haven't eaten in a while, your heart, liver, muscles, kidneys, and brain still require fuel, but where does it come from? In other words, when insulin is not circulating, another hormone or enzyme must be activated to liberate energy. In this case, it's HSL the triglyceride watch guard. HSL is activated during times of low or no fuel and responsible for breaking down triglycerides into individual fats and releasing them into the blood. Individual fats enter the blood and begin supplying your organs and cellular communities with fat calories. Stored triglycerides do serve a purpose as they are used as a source of fuel between meals, while you are sleeping, and during exercise.

Exercise and HSL

During times of prolonged exercise, fats become the preferred fuel. Therefore, storing a bit of fat is normal and healthy, and does get used up. In fact, exercise is the best method of burning fat as it stimulates HSL. Once stimulated, HSL liberates fats into the blood where they travel to your muscles, are burned for energy, and gone forever. Exercising most days of the week keeps HSL active.

Muscles and Sugar Reserves

You may be curious about the "sugar reserves" in your muscles? When are they used? Muscle sugar reserves are used in the early stages of exercise to get the "fire" in your muscles started. The problem is, muscle glycogen doesn't last long. That's where fats come in. Since it will take a short time for fats to arrive at your muscles, sugar reserves must handle the energy obligation. For a short period of time, your muscles will use both glycogen and fats for energy. As exercise duration continues, sugar reserves become depleted, making fats the primary fuel used. The longer you exercise, the longer HSL will continue releasing fats into the blood. Fats are able to supply muscles with fuel for a very long time as there are stock piles of triglycerides available in millions of fat cells.

LPL and Your Muscles

Your muscles are glucose and fat furnaces while your fat cells are fat warehouses. To begin priming you for what takes place in the insulin resistant state, think about what would happen if LPL relocated and permanently started storing triglycerides in your muscles. Would your muscles use fat or glucose as fuel? What would happen to glucose that is stored in your muscles as glycogen? Could your muscles actually hold glycogen and fat, or would these two fuels be separated into different compartments? What if these conditions were to happen to you? Would you be able to notice changes in the way you feel? What would happen to the normal role of insulin? Would more or less be required? Additionally, would your liver, kidneys, and arteries be affected if insulin was no longer able to dictate carbohydrate and fat metabolism?

10 HDL Cholesterol

As attacks on FFC's last for hours creating a mess in the blood, your small intestine and liver decide to help clean up the blood. Each produces a protein, but not the type you eat. Rather, this protein is produced automatically in response to LPL attacks. In other words, specific genes are turned on during dietary fat and cholesterol metabolism which stimulate the production of proteins capable of clearing your blood. This protein is called a1. In the blood, a1 from your small intestine combines with a1 from your liver forming a more complete A1. Newly formed A1 begins collecting triglycerides that escaped the attacks and any triglyceride "remnants" left circulating in the blood post LPL attacks.

The Formation of HDL

Some of the triglycerides that made it back to your liver are placed in a temporary "triglyceride pool". A1, now circulating in the blood begins picking up any cholesterol that never made it to your liver. A1 becomes full of triglycerides, triglyceride remnants, and cholesterol. This maturing process ultimately converts A1 into your "good" or high density lipoprotein (HDL) cholesterol.

Why HDL is "Good" Cholesterol?

Now that you know HDL is not something you eat, you should know why it's your "good" cholesterol. As it travels across miles of arteries acting basically as a garbage truck in your blood, it performs one additional life saving task. It has the unique ability to pick up cholesterol that was previously deposited in your artery lining.

HDL and LCAT

As HDL travels across your arteries keeping them clean, it becomes quite unstable with cholesterol it has collected. To help stabilize HDL for ease of travel, LCAT helps out. LCAT is one assistant assigned to HDL. It is responsible for moving freshly gathered cholesterol into the core of HDL. Moving cholesterol into the center of HDL accomplishes two tasks. It allows for more cholesterol to be picked up from your arteries and it prevents cholesterol from falling out of HDL. HDL eventually heads to your liver to unload this potentially toxic cholesterol.

About Your HDL Cholesterol

There are many factors that adversely affect your HDL cholesterol. For example, aging lowers HDL cholesterol by approximately 1% per year after the age of 50. Weight gain also interferes with HDL cholesterol. In fact, if weight gain leads to pre-diabetes or type II diabetes (insulin resistant states), you're likely to end up with lower than healthy HDL cholesterol. Section two explains this in great detail.

11 The Birth of LDL Cholesterol

While a small amount of glucose is stored as glycogen, excess glucose and all fats entering the liver cannot be permanently stored. If fats or excess glucose that is converted into triglycerides are stored, your liver would become fatty. Even though your liver contains a "triglyceride pool", it's only a temporary holding tank. To prevent fatty liver disease, triglycerides are pulled from the pool, combined with a small amount of cholesterol, a guide, and shipped into the blood. This new compound is called a very low-density lipoprotein or VLDL. VLDL's are extremely rich in triglycerides and contain relatively little cholesterol.

The Release of VLDL

VLDL's are shipped out of your liver into the blood where they are rapidly and violently attacked by none other than LPL, the famous triglyceride thief. Fat cells welcome new fats. With it, they produce and store new triglycerides that serve as a source of future fuel.

From VLDL to LDL

During the attacks on VLDL's, many triglycerides are stolen out of VLDL's, but they retain most of their cholesterol. Some VLDL's do escape the attacks and continue circulating in the blood. What's left is a smaller compound consisting mainly of cholesterol and very little triglyceride.

This new compound full of cholesterol relative to triglycerides is called a low density lipoprotein or LDL.

LDL's Trip Through the Blood

As LDL's circulate, they may become trapped or lodged in stressed areas of your arteries. Their cholesterol is modified and becomes the starting material for heart disease. LDL cholesterol is known as "bad cholesterol" for this exact reason. Some do make it back to your liver where they are removed from the blood. LDL's are not really "bad". They do serve a purpose by delivering cholesterol to cells. They become harmful only if they are left circulating in your arteries or they become trapped in your artery lining.

Dietary Factors That Raise LDL Cholesterol

Saturated fat is one type of dietary fat that raises your LDL cholesterol. It does this by making it very tough for your liver to accept and remove LDL's from circulation. If forced to remain circulating, the greater chance they have of becoming "stuck" in the artery lining.

Trans-fat, which is found in both plant and animal foods is actually worse than saturated fat. It raises LDL cholesterol and lowers HDL cholesterol.

12 HDL's & LDL's

Believe it or not, after HDL's have swept across your arteries extracting potential artery clogging cholesterol, they begin transferring some of their cholesterol. While it seems pro atherogenic to "give up" potentially toxic cholesterol, in the normal and healthy state, HDL's release some of their cholesterol. CETP, the second assistant assigned to HDL, who lives on HDL, is responsible for transferring cholesterol out of HDL.

What Happens To HDL?
HDL's begin "bumping" into VLDL's. While VLDL's are being attacked by LPL and losing triglycerides, they end up gaining some of HDL's cholesterol thanks to CETP. The end result is a VLDL depleted of triglycerides and rich in cholesterol.

HDL's Return to the Liver
HDL's head for the liver to unload any triglycerides and cholesterol not transferred to VLDL's. The triglycerides are sent to the triglyceride pool for temporary holding. They will eventually be incorporated into new VLDL's. Returned cholesterol has two fates. Some will be used to produce bile and some will be temporarily stored.

Fat and Cholesterol Summary

FFC's originate in your intestine from dietary fat and cholesterol. Much of the triglycerides inside FFC's that are released into the blood are stolen by LPL, while dietary cholesterol ends up back at your liver.

VLDL's (very low density lipoproteins) originate in your liver. They also transport fats and a little cholesterol to your cells, but the fats and cholesterol come from your liver, not your diet. Only one fat transporter, FFC or VLDL should be in your blood at any one time under normal conditions.

LDL's originate from VLDL's almost instantly. LDL's are cholesterol transporters, as they acquire this cholesterol. Some of the LDL's end up lodged in your arteries full of cholesterol!

HDL's are also cholesterol transporters, but they remove cholesterol from your blood and arteries. This action of cholesterol transport to the liver for disposal lowers your total blood cholesterol.

BLOOD CHOLESTEROL TABLE

Cholesterol Type	Your Numbers	What Does this Indicate?
LDL Cholesterol	<100	Perfect! Keep them Right Here
	100-129	Pretty Good-Small Changes with Food Choices
	130-159	Too High- Food Strategies restricting Saturated Fat
	160-189	TROUBLE, you need regimented Food Strategies along with regular exercise
	≥ 190	SERIOUS TROUBLE-major league heart disease risk, you'll likely to need medication : (
Total Cholesterol	< 200	Nicely Done
	200-239	Not too Bad, food strategies and weight loss recommended before your doctor wants to put you on medication
	≥ 240	Too High- other than placing blame on genetics, you need to fight and bring it down

Cholesterol Type	Your Numbers	What Does this Indicate?
HDL Cholesterol	<40	Too Low for men-Exercise can bring it up!
	<50	Too Low for women-Exercise can bring it up!
	≥ 60	Great Job-this helps lower your risk of heart disease

Cholesterol is measured in milligrams per deciliter (mg/dl)

The cholesterol table provides you with a gauge of your heart and artery disease risk. Compare these numbers with the numbers from your latest blood work.

LDL is best when it's below 100 mg/dl, total cholesterol is desirable under 200 mg/dl, and HDL, your "good" cholesterol, offers optimal protection above 60 mg/dl. Numbers that fall out of the "healthy" and desirable ranges are likely to be improved through food strategies detailed for you in section four.

13 Energy Regulation

If your car engine gets too hot, a cooling system helps return the temperature back to a safer range. Similarly, if you exercise and begin to heat up your internal (core) temperature, you begin to sweat, which helps cool and return your body temperature back to a safer range. This is regulation at work. If blood sugar becomes temporarily elevated, insulin provides assurance that it will be returned to a normal and desirable range. The opposite is also true. If blood sugar dips too low, your pancreas produces and secretes another hormone capable of increasing blood glucose by converting glycogen into usable glucose. This is the reason your liver stores a bit of glucose as glycogen (sugar reserves)!

Regulation of Fat

The amount of fat circulating in your blood is regulated in several ways. First, dietary fat is regulated by LPL. Triglycerides are stolen by LPL as FFC's circulate throughout your body. LPL's action helps lower the number of FFC's and therefore triglycerides traveling through the blood.

VLDL's, which are also triglyceride transporters, are released from your liver rich in triglycerides only to be depleted by LPL. As triglycerides are stolen by LPL, the result is fewer VLDL's and therefore fewer triglycerides and triglyceride remnants in the blood.

HSL is also involved in regulating how much fat is in your blood. Resting cells such as heart and muscle cells rely on circulating fats for energy. In times of low blood glucose, and therefore low blood insulin, HSL is activated. Stored triglycerides are broken down and released into your blood as individual fats where they are used by heart and muscle cells. Muscle sugar reserves (glycogen) are also regulated by fat. While muscles rely on glycogen, they wait for fats to arrive which supply them with a consistent and seemingly endless supply of calories to be burned. This process helps conserve and therefore regulate glycogen use.

Regulation Summary

These processes just described occur in the *normal state*, with no interruptions in the regulation of carbohydrate or fat metabolism. Insulin and LPL are for lowering blood glucose and fat, while glycogen and HSL are involved in increasing blood glucose and fat levels respectively. Together they help maintain a normal range of fuel at all times keeping your blood healthy and balanced.

SECTION II

THE INSULIN RESISTANT STATE

14 Abnormal Blood Glucose

What if insulin lost its stimulatory and inhibitory features and no longer had the ability to regulate blood glucose and fat? For example, what if insulin wasn't powerful enough to stimulate fat cells to dispose of excess glucose? What if insulin wasn't powerful enough to stimulate muscle cells to dispose of glucose? What if insulin was no longer able to suppress your liver's release of glucose? Where would all of this glucose go? Would your pancreas be forced to work overtime? Would all of the excess insulin be harmful?

If you have "high blood sugar" you better take action. It means these events along with other heart and artery disease events are unfolding. If you let these early stages of insulin resistance progress, expect high blood pressure and artery damage, elevated triglycerides, and low levels of protective HDL cholesterol. In fact, you may never develop type II diabetes, but you will experience heart attack promoting states along the way.

What Causes Insulin Resistance?

Weight gain is perhaps the main link between normal glucose disposal and inefficient glucose disposal. Insulin resistance is the diminished effectiveness of insulin to stimulate your cells. If your cells are less responsive to insulin, they have become glucose intolerant. This is why you end up with higher than normal blood glucose levels. A simple blood test will indicate to what extent your cells have become less responsive to insulin. Currently, there are two tests, the impaired fasting glucose (IFG) and oral glucose tolerance test (OGTT). Both detect states of abnormal blood glucose control.

Impaired Fasting Glucose (IFG)

In a fasted state, usually 12 hours, normal blood glucose levels should be less than 100 mg per deciliter (mg/dl). If the results show blood glucose between 100 mg/dl and less than 126 mg/dl, you're insulin resistant and suffering from impaired fasting glucose (IFG). At this stage, you are pre-diabetic. Specifically, the IFG test indicates liver insulin resistance or the inability of insulin to regulate glucose production and release. If your IFG test reads higher than 126 mg/dl, you would be classified as a type two diabetic.

Oral Glucose Tolerance Test (OGTT)

The oral glucose tolerance test (OGTT) test is similar to the IFG test. It tests your blood glucose two hours after you have consumed a "sugary liquid". Normal or healthy and acceptable blood glucose levels following this test should be no higher than 140 mg/dl of blood glucose. Greater than 140 mg/dl but less than 200 mg/dl of blood glucose indicates impaired glucose tolerance (IGT) or pre-diabetes. This means insulin resistance is occurring at your muscles in addition to your liver. At 200 mg/dl or greater, you would be classified as a diabetic.

Current recommendations are to have the IFG test done first followed by the 2 hour OGTT the following day. This process allows physicians to see the severity of your insulin resistant state and specifically where it is occurring.

The Difference Between Pre-Diabetes and Type II Diabetes

In order for type II diabetes to develop, three criteria must be met. First, your cells are severely insulin resistant as they are no longer responding to insulin stimulation. Second, your pancreas is damaged to the point where it produces inefficient concentrations of insulin. This helps explain why your cells are unable to dispose of glucose. Third, glucose intolerance becomes evident as insulin resistance of your liver

What State Do You Live In?

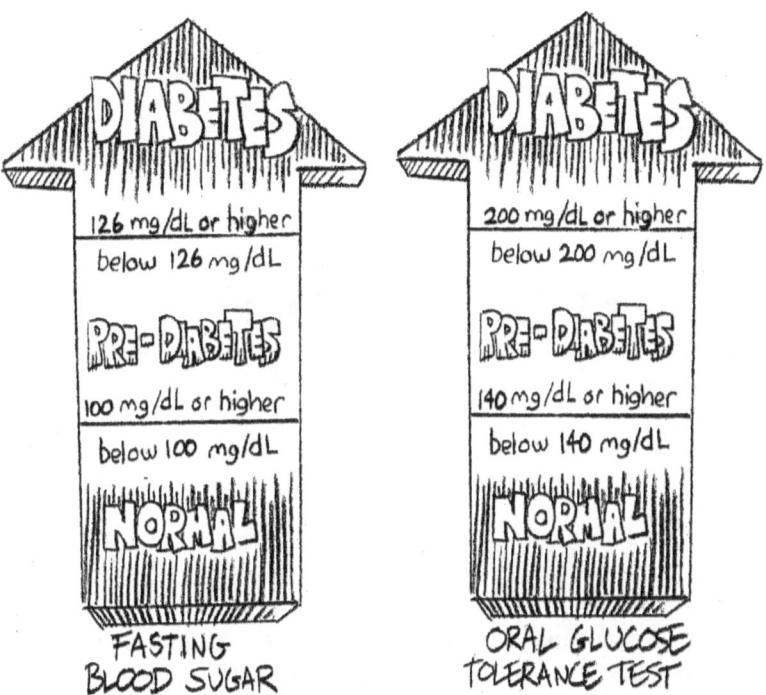

The IFG and OGTT determine the severity of your weight related insulin resistant state.

and muscles (whole body insulin resistance) produces sustained high blood glucose or hyperglycemia. Without medications, blood glucose remains toxic.

With pre-diabetes, only one criterion is required, insulin resistance. The pre-diabetic state means your pancreas is still functioning at a level where it produces and secretes enough insulin to stimulate and overpower the resistance of your cells. This extra pressure by insulin forces cells to open and dispose of glucose. This alleviates the hyperglycemic state. Unfortunately, this temporary hyperglycemic state does progress if left untreated. It promotes high blood pressure, elevated triglycerides, low HDL cholesterol, and toxic levels of insulin, all leading up to full blown type II diabetes.

15 Fat Compartments

Body fat can appear just about anywhere, but the areas most recognizable are the hips, thighs, and especially the stomach. Stomach fat, the type you can see is called subcutaneous fat. There are many names given to this type of fat. It is called apple shaped fat, android fat, beer belly fat, cardiac fat, central fat, paunch fat, mid-section fat, and truncal fat. It's the layer of fat you can pinch as it lies between your skin and muscles. Subcutaneous fat compartments take years to fill. If they become large enough, they split into two new smaller fat cells capable of growing into mature fat cells. This process repeats itself for decades. At some point, subcutaneous fat cells reach a threshold and divert excess calories to a secondary fat storage area called visceral fat.

Visceral Fat

You can't see or pinch visceral fat as it lies underneath subcutaneous fat. It develops on top and around your organs. Visceral fat acts similar to subcutaneous fat in two ways. It too takes in excess calories where they are converted and stored as triglycerides. You can also find LPL, the triglyceride thief located on visceral fat cells. The main difference between the two lies in the way visceral fat behaves if you develop weight related insulin resistance.

Insulin Resistance and Hyperglycemia

During insulin resistance, glucose shows up outside the cell, but normal insulin concentrations are too weak to stimulate fat cells to dispose of excess glucose. This results in temporary hyperglycemia as glucose is forced to remain outside your cells in the blood.

Insulin Resistance and Hyperinsulinemia

Your pancreas is in a state of emergency. With fat cells not fully responding to insulin, blood glucose levels continue escalating. Your pancreas begins producing and shipping even more insulin into the blood. This overproduction of insulin, and there's quite a bit being released into the blood, alleviates hyperglycemia by forcing your cells open. Blood glucose and insulin levels do return to normal, but not for long as your weight related insulin resistant state continuously promotes this vicious cycle. Your body has paid a dear price. Your pancreas has been forced to work overtime and your arteries have been subjected to excessive levels of insulin, a condition known as hyperinsulinemia. While the hyperglycemic and hyperinsulinemic states are temporary in the early stages of insulin resistance, the problem is, you can't feel the destruction they're causing.

Insulin Resistance and Fats Escaping Into The Blood

As a result of excess blood insulin, HSL, the triglyceride guard who lives in your fat cells is awakened. HSL begins breaking down triglycerides and releasing individual fats into the blood. Some fats make their way into your liver which now begins dealing with this influx and attempts to prevent their accumulation. First, it "burns" some of the fats. Next, your liver begins converting fats into triglycerides and storing them in the triglyceride pool. Unfortunately, neither approach lasts very long as fats from millions of fat cells begin to infiltrate your liver.

Problems for Your Liver

Fats entering your liver begin interrupting insulin's normal suppressive effects on glucose production and release. In the insulin resistant state, liver glycogen (sugar reserves) is broken down and released into the blood creating higher blood glucose. To make matters worse, some of the fats entering your liver are converted into "new" glucose. This glucose is shipped into the blood creating even higher blood glucose. The hyperglycemic state is in full effect as glucose production from glycogen breakdown along with new glucose results in the hyperglycemic state. As a result of blood glucose overload, your pancreas begins working as hard as it can to produce and ship insulin into the blood to normalize your hyperglycemic condition.

Exercise, Insulin Resistance, and HSL

One of the best ways to stop HSL from releasing fats into the blood is to stop insulin surges. There are a few ways to accomplish this.

First, begin exercising. While it may sound extremely general, any type of exercise for a short period of time each day will help inactivate HSL by lowering blood insulin concentrations. How does this happen? Exercise not only burns calories, which frees up room in fat cells, it causes cells to "open up" without insulin stimulation. If cells begin to dispose of glucose without insulin stimulation, blood insulin concentrations improve. The lower your blood insulin, the less active is HSL. It's a win win situation for you as you're improving the hyperglycemic and hyperinsulinemic state by shutting off the release of fats into the blood.

Diet, Insulin Resistance, and HSL

Omega 3 fats found in coldwater fish such as salmon, tuna, trout, and mackerel help prevent unwanted HSL activity. How much and how often you should you consume these protein sources is planned for you in the food strategies section.

16 Insulin Resistance & High Blood Fats

The triglyceride pool is becoming too large as the influx of fats entering your liver is endless. In an effort to prevent fatty liver disease, your liver begins shipping large quantities of triglycerides into the blood. Of course the triglycerides have to be shipped inside a transporter. To accomplish this, your liver produces a new compound that consists of mainly triglycerides, a little cholesterol, and a guide. This compound is a very low density lipoprotein (VLDL). It's the same VLDL you were introduced to in the normal state. The difference is, in the insulin resistant state, masses of VLDL's are being produced and released into the blood thanks to increased HSL activity.

Insulin Resistance, Dietary Fat, and Hypertriglyceridemia

Consuming dietary fat complicates matters even further. With overwhelming concentrations of blood insulin (hyperinsulinemia), LPL attacks are delayed. The result is hyper blood levels of fats or hypertriglyceridemia. The triglycerides come from those that escaped FFC and VLDL attacks plus fats leaking from fat cells. Your blood is toxic as it's full of triglycerides. As these sources of triglycerides make their way into your liver, it has no choice but to produce and ship them back into the blood inside VLDL's!

Carbohydrates Make It Worse

Consuming carbohydrates, regardless of their "good" or "bad" identity, adds to your hyperglycemic and hypertriglyceridemic state. Glucose from digested carbohydrates cannot be used by your liver since it's insulin resistant. Instead, glucose entering the blood is considered to be excess and is dealt with in two ways. First, some glucose will be rejected and forced back into your blood. This exacerbates your hyperglycemic state. This is why your blood glucose soars each time you consume carbohydrate. Second, glucose that does make it into your liver will be converted into triglycerides and stored in the triglyceride pool. The pool is at maximum capacity and your liver has no choice but to ship more VLDL's into the blood.

NORMAL TRIGLYCERIDES	< 150 mg/dl
BORDERLINE HIGH TRIGLYCERIDES	150-199 mg/dl
HIGH TRIGLYCERIDES	200-499 mg/dl
VERY HIGH TRIGLYCERIDES	> 500 mg/dl

Triglycerides are measured in milligrams per deciliter (mg/dl)

You Can Lower High Triglycerides

If your triglycerides are higher than 150 mg/dl, which is considered to be the upper acceptable limit, your risk of developing heart and artery disease increases. The higher they rise, the greater your risk. With very high blood triglycerides, your chances of developing pancreatitis or inflammation of the pancreas, is significant. Omega 3 fatty acids, which are found in coldwater fish and a few types of nuts, seeds, and oils, can help lower blood triglycerides by;
- Helping your liver burn triglycerides
- Preventing triglyceride storage
- Enhancing the production of liver glycogen, a sign of a healthy liver
- Speeding up the dissolution of VLDL's being produced in your liver
- Reducing the secretion of VLDL's into the blood

Plant Omega 3's

Plant sources of omega 3's are scarce and include walnuts, flaxseeds, and canola oil. Olive oil is a relatively poor source. While many foods in the supermarket may be rich in omega 3's, beware, as the source of these omega fats may not provide you with the same triglyceride lowering effectiveness as fish omega 3's. Plant omega 3's are found in the form of alpha-linolenic acid, commonly known as ALA. In the body, ALA is converted into the two popular fish omega 3's, eicosapentaenoic (EPA) and docosahexaenoic (DHA) acid. The issue with plant omega 3's is that less than 5% of the ALA they contain is converted into EPA and DHA. Don't get caught up in buying omega 3 fortified eggs, mayonnaise, yogurts, or cereals for the sole purpose of reducing high blood triglycerides. But don't throw away the walnuts and flaxseeds just yet. They have many powerful qualities that improve weight related insulin resistant conditions such as high blood glucose and high blood pressure. All six levels of food strategies in section four provide you with both plant and fish sources of omega 3 fats.

17 Insulin Resistance & Lower HDL Cholesterol

The insulin resistant state begins taking a toll on your HDL cholesterol. With massive amounts of VLDL's being released into the blood, HDL's are adversely impacted in two ways. First, HDL's become smaller in size as they are forced to transfer their cholesterol to VLDL's. Second, smaller HDL's cannot remain circulating in the blood. Your liver begins extracting these now less effective cholesterol transporters. Fewer and smaller circulating HDL's contribute to the development of atherosclerosis as they are less able to gather cholesterol from your artery lining.

Raising HDL Levels

If you're insulin resistant and suffer from low HDL cholesterol, the question becomes, how do you raise your numbers to a protective level? Two of the best non-pharmacological ways to improve HDL is through exercise and weight loss.

Exercise and HDL Cholesterol

Exercise helps slow CETP activity, the assistant who lives on HDL and is responsible for transferring cholesterol out of HDL. With less cholesterol traded out of HDL, they remain a bit larger in size which keeps them circulating. The longer they circulate, the more cholesterol they pick up from your artery lining.

Exercise duration and frequency also contribute to healthy HDL levels. As a general rule of thumb, walking or jogging 20 miles per week or expending at least 1,200 calories over a five day period improves HDL cholesterol. Additionally, the weight loss you achieve through exercise can further improve your HDL levels by up to 5%.

Increasing HDL Cholesterol With Food

It's very difficult to improve HDL with food alone, but adding red pepper and garlic to your diet may slow cholesterol loss out of HDL. If HDL's retain their cholesterol, they're less likely to be taken out of circulation.

18 Insulin Resistance & Your Muscles

Another consequence of becoming insulin resistant is the relocation of LPL, the triglyceride thief who normally resides on fat cells. The next cellular community where LPL establishes residency is your muscles. For a while, fats entering your muscles can be burned up, but this doesn't last long as fats enter at uncontrollable rates. Unlike your liver, which can temporarily store some fat in the triglyceride pool, your muscles do not have this luxury. Your muscles become confused as they cannot handle the influx of fats while they metabolize glucose. The result is slowed glucose uptake and halted glycogen production.

Impaired Glucose Tolerance (IGT)

The accumulation of triglycerides inside your muscles is a sign of advanced insulin resistance and a likely sign of type II diabetes. A few serious consequences result. First, you end up with advanced hyperglycemia or whole body insulin resistance as muscles account for the majority of glucose disposal. Second, as you're unable to build and maintain adequate muscle glycogen, fatigue sets in very quickly during basic activities and exercise.

You have come full circle on IFG and IGT. Impaired fasting glucose (IFG) represents insulin resistance at the level of your liver and IGT represents insulin resistance at the level of your muscles. Insulin resistance of this severity is likely to have caused extensive artery and pancreas damage.

Top Twelve Reasons Exercise Improves Insulin Resistance

1. Exercise burns blood glucose which improves the hyperglycemic state.
2. Exercise helps dispose glucose without insulin stimulation.
3. Exercise helps muscles rebuild glycogen stores, which improves whole body insulin resistance.
4. Exercise increases the amount of insulin traveling across your arteries which increases glucose uptake into your cells.
5. Exercise improves blood circulation in distal areas of your body such as your fingers and toes.
6. Exercise lowers blood triglycerides, which improves the hypertriglyceridemic state.
7. Exercise reduces the accumulation of fats within your muscles.
8. Exercise improves LPL activity, a sign of improved insulin resistance.
9. Exercise improves your "good" or HDL cholesterol.
10. Exercise burns stored fat, shrinking fat cells.
11. Exercise inhibits HSL from releasing fats into the blood.
12. Exercise lowers blood pressure.

19 Your Toxic Blood

The overweight state has promoted the insulin resistant state. The insulin resistant state has produced several unwanted hyper states. These include the states of glycemia, triglyceridemia, and insulinemia. As a result, your liver, pancreas, and muscles are being destroyed. But what about your blood, what does it look like? Imagine how polluted it must be from years worth of *excess* glucose, *excess* fats, and *excess* insulin. Throw in cholesterol rich LDL's and your blood is really a toxic river running across your arteries. It's hard to clean up a mess like this especially when the insulin resistant state produces fewer HDL's. Your time line is shrinking. The insulin resistant state is in full swing and a heart attack is on the horizon.

Your Pancreas and Insulin Resistance

Your pancreas is always producing insulin. Even in times of low blood glucose or when you're sleeping, it's producing and shipping some insulin into the blood. This minimal amount of insulin is protective, but the insulin resistant state changes this. Excessive fats leaking into the blood create two threatening scenarios. First, they produce free radicals, which can be thought of as molecules capable of destroying and killing cells. Second, fats eventually make their way into your pancreas where they stimulate the production and release of more insulin. If fat leakage from fat cells is not stopped, the pancreas will eventually burn out. If you let this occur, you will be forced into the diabetic and medicated state.

20 High Blood Pressure

One third of all adults in America have high blood pressure or hypertension, a more severe form of high blood pressure. Even if you have normal blood pressure as an adult, you have a 90% chance of developing hypertension in your lifetime. Before exploring the relationship between weight related insulin resistance and blood pressure, you need to understand your arteries and the pressure of blood inside them.

What is Blood Pressure?

Your arteries act as fuel lines or conduits that deliver blood components such as nutrients, chemicals, hormones, water, cells, and oxygen to all cells in your body. They also float triglyceride and cholesterol transporters such as FFC's, VLDL's, LDL's, and HDL's. As blood flows against the inner walls of your arteries, it creates pressure, just like water flowing through a garden hose creates pressure on the inside of the hose. Ideally, you want to keep your arteries as clean and debris free as possible, as any "artery traffic" will interfere with blood flow leading to blood pressure issues. The easier and smoother it is for blood components to flow across your arteries, your risk of high blood pressure is significantly reduced.

How is Blood Pressure Measured?

Blood pressure is measured using a cuff called a sphygmomanometer.

It is placed around your arm and measures the amount of pressure in one of the large arteries in your arm. If blood pressure is higher than normal in this artery, you can be sure that pressure is even greater near your heart, where the force of blood originates.

Special Features of Your Arteries

Your arteries are capable of handling large fluctuations in blood volume or blood pressure. The muscularity and elasticity features of your arteries allow them to expand and contract on an "as needed basis". These features prevent high blood pressure. For example, exercise may cause a sudden increase in blood pressure. As your heart rate increases, more blood is pumped through your arteries. The arteries handle this increased pressure of blood by expanding. Shortly after exercise is complete, arteries will recoil back into their original shape thanks to these special features. Additionally, muscular and elastic arteries, which are a sign of healthy arteries, aren't as easily "stretched out" from the added pressure of blood forced through them. Just imagine how many times throughout your life your arteries have had to respond to blood pressure increases!

Unique Function of Your Artery Lining

Besides their special features, the question becomes, if arteries are muscular, elastic, and able to expand and contract as needed, how do they know when to do this?

Your entire artery lining is made up of special cells called endothelial cells. These cells join together to form one long smooth surface called the endothelium. This surface creates the perfect highway for blood traffic. Endothelial cells produce "signals" for your arteries to open or close, allowing for controllable changes in blood pressure. With your artery lining being 60,000 miles long, that's quite a few special cells capable of producing and sending the open or close signal. Nitric oxide is the signal. It's actually a gas produced by healthy endothelial cells that prevents high blood pressure. No matter where the artery starts, near your heart, or ends, in distant places like your fat or muscle cells, this lining is known as the endothelium. The only difference in the artery is that the further it travels from your heart, the thinner it becomes.

High Blood Pressure

High blood pressure begins when your systolic pressure (top number) reaches 140 mg/dl *or* your diastolic pressure (bottom number) reaches 90 mg/dl. Either one categorizes you as having advancing and unhealthy blood pressure.

Hypertension and Pre-Hypertension

Hypertension is synonymous with high blood pressure. It is advancing blood pressure of systolic or diastolic pressure or both at rest. Stage one and two are the main hypertensive states, known as primary or essential hypertension. Don't ignore pre-hypertension. It's also a state of hypertension that calls for immediate attention as it acts as a warning sign to stage I hypertension.

BLOOD PRESSURE	SYSTOLIC (TOP NUMBER)	DIASTOLIC (BOTTOM NUMBER)
Normal	<120 &	<80
Pre-hypertension	120-139 or	80-89
Stage 1 Hypertension	140-159 or	90-99
Stage II Hypertension	160+ or	100+

Blood pressure is measured in millimeters of mercury per deciliter (mm Hg/dl)

Causes of High Blood Pressure

There are many contributing causes of high blood pressure. Uncontrollable causes include aging and genetics. Controllable causes include smoking, excessive drinking, physical inactivity, diet inadequacy, and weight gain. All of these blood pressure raising "risk factors" share a common end result, which is damage to the surface (endothelium) of your arteries.

Weight Gain and High Blood Pressure

Weight gain is the single most controllable cause of high blood pressure. Blood pressure is proportional to your body weight. If your weight goes up, so does blood pressure. If your weight comes down, so does blood pressure. With weight gain, problems begin when your heart needs to pump harder and faster, with more force, to keep up with your oversized state. The extra demand placed on your heart as a result of excess body mass results in high blood pressure as each heart beat ejects a greater volume of blood into circulation.

The Smallest Arteries

Arteries traveling to distant places like your eyes, fat cells, fingers, and toes, are much thinner compared to arteries near your heart. Arteries that deliver blood into these remote areas are called capillaries. They are so small and thin that the hormone insulin is just able to squeeze through. As insulin travels through these spider web thin arteries, it's able to stimulate the endothelium to begin producing nitric oxide. Not only does it activate endothelial cells to produce the signal, it prepares endothelial cells for incoming nutrients. The only problem with having a microscopic diameter is that capillaries are very susceptible to blood pressure fluctuations.

Insulin Resistance, Artery Dysfunction, and Hypertension

Any damage to the endothelium results in high blood pressure. Damaged endothelial cells become dysfunctional resulting in decreased nitric oxide production. Without this signal, arteries do not open and close as they should. In the insulin resistant state, the hyperglycemic and hypertriglyceridemic states have produced free radicals which destroy all cells, including endothelial cells. As long as weight related insulin resistant states persist, endothelial cells will continue to be destroyed resulting in decreased nitric oxide production and eventually hypertension. The situation worsens. The hyperinsulinemic cycles you're experiencing increase the amount of sodium your kidneys reabsorb. This creates greater blood volume, greater demand on your heart, and high blood pressure! As endothelial cells in capillaries become damaged, peripheral artery disease (PAD) or peripheral vascular disease (PVD) is a likely consequence.

Exercise, Artery Health, and Hypertension

Exercise falls into one of two categories, aerobic or anaerobic. Aerobic exercise requires oxygen while anaerobic can be performed for short periods of time without oxygen. Both types improve blood pressure and both should be part of your daily regimen. For example, aerobic exercise such as brisk walking or light jogging "stresses" your endothelium (endothelial cells) to produce nitric oxide. Similarly, weight lifting, the anaerobic portion of your daily exercise routine not only stimulates muscles to devour body fat, your lower body weight results in lower blood pressure.

Nutrition, Artery Health, and Hypertension

While no single nutrient is solely responsible for improving weight related insulin resistant hypertension, there are several that will improve artery function and collectively reverse hypertension. Nutrients such as calcium, magnesium, potassium, and folate rich foods offer blood pressure improving properties. Add in foods full of fiber and healthy unsaturated fats such as mufas and pufas, and you can expect improved blood pressure. By the way, never add salt to any of your meals or snacks. Sodium is found naturally in most foods and by day's end, you will have consumed plenty of this mineral without the need or benefit to add additional salt. Adding salt to food creates more blood volume, which results in further blood pressure surges. By far, sodium is the most over consumed nutrient in our daily diet. The food strategies in section four provide you with foods full of nutrients that minimize sodium intake and promote sodium elimination.

21 The Metabolic Syndrome

For decades upon decades, heart and artery disease was thought to be caused by or linked to a single condition such as type II diabetes, hypertension, obesity, a high fat diet, or abnormal blood cholesterol. You never heard of cardiovascular disease being caused by more than one or several chronic disease states. Today, we know different. We know that your risk of developing heart and artery disease is much greater if you suffer from multiple co-existing conditions. This is the metabolic syndrome or what used to be called the insulin resistance syndrome. It's a cluster or group of chronic disease states that stem from being insulin resistant. The consequences of the metabolic syndrome raise your risk of heart and artery disease by nearly 200% and type II diabetes by nearly 500%.

The entire story I have developed to this point is the story of the metabolic syndrome. It starts when weight gain leads to insulin resistance and progresses well beyond "high blood glucose". If the insulin resistant state is not controlled with food and exercise, it's likely that you'll end up with at least one other dysmetabolic state such as abnormal blood pressure, blood cholesterol, or blood triglycerides. Being informed that your are suffering from pre-diabetes or high blood pressure or low HDL cholesterol is upsetting in itself, but imagine if you're overweight and living with several heart attack promoting conditions.

Jerrod P. Libonati, MS, RD

The Criteria

There are a total of five criteria (individual risk factors) that make up the metabolic syndrome. They include obesity, impaired fasting glucose (insulin resistance), elevated triglycerides, hypertension, and low HDL cholesterol. Living with any three, and in no particular order, would label you with having the metabolic syndrome.

Criteria 1: Waist Circumference

For men, if your waist circumference reaches 102 cm (centimeters) or 40 inches, you're obese. For women, don't let your waist circumference reach 88 cm or 35 inches as you'll be classified as clinically obese. If you become obese, your risk of developing type II diabetes and artery disease is significantly increased. Currently, one third or approximately 33% of adults are obese or approximately thirty pounds or more overweight.

Criteria 2: Elevated Blood Glucose

It all started when your fat cells became resistant to insulin. Fats began trickling into the blood and eventually into your liver. Not only did these fats impair insulin action in your liver, they began promoting the production and release of glucose into the blood, further raising your blood glucose. If either test, the impaired fasting glucose or the oral glucose tolerance test indicates higher than normal blood glucose, you're insulin resistant. If you're obese and insulin resistant, you not only meet two criteria required for classification under the metabolic syndrome, your risk of heart and artery disease increases by 150%.

Criteria 3: High Triglycerides

While obesity shows great association with insulin resistance, being overweight and insulin resistant is the strongest link to high blood triglycerides. In the insulin resistant state, not only are fats being released from stomach fat cells, there are tremendous concentrations of triglyceride transporters such as VLDL's and FFC's circulating in the blood that contribute to unhealthy blood fat levels. Collectively, blood triglycerides will end up higher than 150 mg/dl, classifying you with hypertriglyceridemia and increasing your odds of suffering a heart attack. It also adds to your growing number of metabolic syndrome criteria. As long as you remain at least overweight, as defined by your waist circumference, and insulin resistant, your fat compartments will continue to release fats into the blood.

Criteria 4: Low HDL Cholesterol

Low levels of HDL cholesterol, less than 40 mg/dl in men and less than 50 mg/dl in women are not only independent contributors towards heart and artery disease, low HDL cholesterol is linked with high blood triglycerides. Not only are there fewer circulating HDL's in the insulin resistant state, they are smaller in size and therefore less cardio protective. If you are at least overweight and suffering from unhealthy triglycerides, chances are, you'll end up with small and insufficient quantities of HDL cholesterol, further raising your risk of heart and artery disease.

Criteria 5: High Blood Pressure

Heart attack and stroke risk is increased when systolic blood pressure reaches 140 *or* diastolic blood pressure reads 90. *Either one* indicates high blood pressure. As long as the overweight and obese states continue to escalate, so will blood pressure. Pre-hypertension is one of the most common signs of the metabolic syndrome as it likely indicates your body weight is too high. Don't ignore its potential. If your blood pressure is high, you have met another criterion of the metabolic syndrome.

METABOLIC SYNDROME COMPONENTS

CRITERIA	CUT OFF POINT	SEX
WAIST CIRCUMFERENCE	> 40 INCHES OR 102 CM	MEN
	> 35 INCHES OR 88 CM	WOMEN
TRIGYLCERIDES	≥ 150	MEN AND WOMEN
HIGH DENSITY LIPOPROTEIN (HDL)	< 40 < 50	MEN WOMEN

CRITERIA	CUT OFF POINT	SEX
BLOOD PRESSURE	≥ 130 / ≥ 85	MEN AND WOMEN
FASTING BLOOD GLUCOSE	≥ 100	MEN AND WOMEN

Fasting blood sugar is defined by IFG or IGT;
Impaired Fasting Glucose (IFG) Impaired Glucose Tolerance (IGT)
Metabolic Syndrome as defined by the National Cholesterol Education Program (NCEP) Adult Treatment Panel III (ATP III).

Reversing The Metabolic Syndrome

There is no single cure for the metabolic syndrome. The optimal way to approach this cumulative metabolic disorder is to lose weight using specific foods and their nutrients. Just as important as the quality of your foods is the spacing of your calories, the current ratio of nutrients at snacks and meals, and preventing calorie peaks and valleys. All of this has been planned for you in the food strategies section.

22 Heart Disease

The arteries lying across your heart, the coronary arteries are the blood vessels most susceptible to heart disease. As your heart receives nutrients by way of the coronary arteries, they are at great risk of becoming extremely damaged as the insulin resistant state promotes toxic levels of glucose, fats, triglycerides, cholesterol rich LDL's, and free radicals. Your blood is toxic. What a mess, and it all started with your overweight state. Let's examine how the insulin resistant state has promoted heart disease.

The Immune Response

As LDL's transport cholesterol across your arteries they undergo structural changes brought about by your toxic blood. These changes create something called oxidized LDL's and promote their accumulation within damaged areas of your coronary arteries. This activates your immune system. Your immune system begins releasing immune cells called monocytes.

Monocytes

Monocytes are like cookie monsters. They dive into your artery lining hunting for oxidized cholesterol rich LDL's. Once monocytes are inside the lining interior, they begin devouring oxidized LDL's. They gorge themselves on LDL's until they're so full, they turn into foam cells.

Foam Cells

Problems arise for foam cells as they become so swollen with cholesterol they are forced back to the surface of your artery. Welcome to the atherosclerotic state as this cholesterol rich foam cell gets half stuck. Part of it remains in the interior of your artery lining and the other half becomes plaque on the endothelium. The plaque not only damages your artery lining (endothelial dysfunction), thereby decreasing nitric oxide production and raising blood pressure, it inhibits the inner layer of artery cells from receiving their nutrients. Without nutrients, cells die. Your artery wall begins to breakdown as more cells starve. Scarring occurs around dead cells and the surrounding areas which become stiff and rigid. Tone and elasticity is lost and arteries are no longer able to recoil back into their original shape. Welcome to the advanced hypertensive state. As long as weight related insulin resistant states continue, you should expect these recurring events.

SECTION III

THE GREAT DIET DEBATE

23 Reversing Weight Related Insulin Resistance

You are suffering from weight related insulin resistance and decide to take action. Before developing a plan, there are many general questions you begin asking yourself. For example, how many calories should I eat? How many times each day should I eat? What about snacking, will it hurt or help me? Is it best not to snack? Will I be forced to give up everything I love to eat and drink? Will I have to commit to strenuous exercise? As you begin to research and design your strategy, specific questions begin to surface. Is there are a single "best" approach to treat weight related insulin resistance? What if I have the metabolic syndrome? Which condition deserves priority and how will I manage the others? What is the optimal ratio of carbs, protein, and fat for treating weight related insulin resistance? How will I be able to lower my blood pressure when sodium is found in nearly all foods? Should I be taking a specific supplement?

The true and big picture of using real food and exercise strategies to reverse weight related insulin resistant states becomes lost as you're bombarded with hundreds of food choices, fad diets, conflicting opinions, myths, and the recent surge of anti-oxidant drinks that pretty much claim to save your life.

There are two schools of theory used to treat and manage the types of heart and artery diseases caused by your state of weight. Research from around the world is still quite controversial regarding the low-fat versus the low-carb approach in treating, reversing, and managing weight related insulin resistance. There are pros and cons of each. In trying to determine if one is more "optimal" that the other, that will be for you to decide as my concluding remarks are likely to startle you. Let's start with the most traditional approach in treating weight related insulin resistance, a low-fat diet.

24 Lower Fat Diets & Insulin Resistance

It's been known for decades that diets rich in total and saturated fat along with dietary cholesterol raise your risk of heart and artery disease. Will a food strategy that is controlled for dietary fat and dietary cholesterol improve weight related insulin resistance and other co-existing conditions?

The claims of a traditional lower fat higher carb diet to reverse weight related insulin resistance and reduce heart and artery disease risk include;
- Lower fat diets improve insulin resistance
- Lower fat diets help lower total and LDL cholesterol
- Lower fat diets improve artery health and reduce blood pressure
- Lower fat diets are rich in anti-oxidants

Lower Fat Diets Improve Insulin Resistance

Lower fat means fiber, vitamin and mineral, and anti-oxidant rich carbs. Carbs that meet these criteria are "good" carbs. They include complex carbs such as vegetables, beans and legumes, and whole grain bread, rice, and pastas. Other good carbs include simple carbs such as fruit, milk, and yogurt. These carbs are exactly what the fat and cholesterol experts were trying to relay to us to eat in place of foods rich in dietary fat and cholesterol. When fat free and lower fat foods were introduced, that's when we became confused. If you need good carbs to reverse weight related insulin resistant states, then fat free pretzels, cookies, and ice cream were not the types recommended in place of dietary fat and cholesterol. When we were told to follow a lower fat diet to reduce heart and artery disease risk, we took it to the extreme. Instructions on how to properly implement a lower fat food strategy were blown out of proportion. We obviously forgot about the simple calories in versus calories out equation as it relates to weight gain. Decades later, we are larger than ever and with more annual cases of heart and artery disease. Ask yourself, "was my weight gain caused by overeating carbs, or was it caused by simply eating too many calories? The answer is obvious. I am sure the statement "consume nearly half of your total daily calories from carbohydrates" scares you, especially with all the hype surrounding low-carb diets. The truth is, if you consume lower fat, high fiber, vitamin and mineral rich carbs, it's "healthfully easy" to eat 40-60% of your total daily calories from carbs without increasing your risk of weight gain, insulin resistance, or cardiovascular disease.

There are two fat free carbohydrate exceptions you should include as part of the optimal plan to fight insulin resistance, milk and yogurt. For about 100 calories, these two carbs provide you with calcium, magnesium, potassium, vitamin A, vitamin D, and the B-vitamin riboflavin. Collectively, they provide essential nutrients, anti-oxidants, and promote healthy blood vessels.

In fact, "good" carbs help reverse insulin resistance by promoting weight loss. Replacing equal portions of fat calories with good carb calories results in fewer total calories consumed. Presto, the caloric deficit over time leads to weight loss. Weight loss improves insulin resistance by "freeing up space" in your fat cells. This allows insulin to effectively direct excess calories into storage. The result is improved blood glucose! Some of these lower fat carbs may even be slightly high in sugar, but don't stress about the sugar content. You won't lose control of your blood glucose if you eat *a piece* of fruit, have a *half cup* of starchy vegetables like beans, peas, potatoes, or drink an *8 fluid ounce* glass of milk. If the portion is controlled, so are glucose and insulin concentrations as both rise in proportion to the *quantity* consumed. Eat a little carb, expect a little rise in blood glucose and blood insulin levels, plain and simple.

Good carbs, like vegetables, fruit, and whole grains are high in fiber. These extremely lower fat foods help manage insulin resistance as fiber minimizes blood glucose surges. Additionally, many good carbs are high in water. The high water content of "good" carbs is appreciated by your cellular communities such as your muscles, liver, and kidneys as all are actively involved in nutrient trafficking. The high water content of these "good carbs" also keeps you hydrated! Lower fat carbs are planned for you in all six levels of food strategies in section four.

Lower Fat Diets and Improved Total and LDL Cholesterol

The most well known feature of a traditional lower fat diet is its effect on improving total and LDL cholesterol. Consuming fiber rich complex carbs in place of fat calories improves your blood cholesterol in several ways.

The simplest way to improve blood cholesterol is to consume less dietary cholesterol. With less dietary cholesterol entering the blood, less ends up in your liver where it's ultimately shipped back into your blood.

The second way to lower blood cholesterol is to eat less dietary fat. With less fat entering the blood, less reaches your liver. This keeps a lid on cholesterol production as "fat fragments" are one ingredient in cholesterol production. With less produced, less will be shipped into the blood. This results in lower total blood cholesterol.

Eating fiber rich lower fat carbs is a third way to lower your total blood cholesterol. Oats, oat bran, peas, oranges, apples, and carrots contain soluble fiber. There are other sources, but the point is, soluble fiber not only delays glucose absorption, it binds to dietary cholesterol. Once bound to cholesterol, the fiber-cholesterol compound is eliminated from your body. This action lowers your total blood cholesterol. Other non-carbohydrate sources of soluble fiber that have the same effect include nuts and seeds. You just have to make sure you exercise portion control as the caloric content of nuts and seeds add up quick.

Reducing saturated fat (sat fat) is the best method to lower your total and LDL cholesterol. Saturated fat negatively impacts your LDL cholesterol by preventing your liver from removing cholesterol rich LDL's from the blood.

Consuming foods with saturated fat also promotes the production of VLDL's, those triglyceride transporters. As more are produced, more will be released into the blood. The issue becomes unfortunate as the insulin resistant state speeds up the conversion of VLDL's to LDL's. One of the surest ways to keep saturated fat intake as low as possible is to consume foods found in your food portfolio listed in section four.

Lower Fat Diets, Improved Artery Health, and Blood Pressure

There are other notable features of consuming a lower fat diet. Overall, it's likely to be low in sodium. Fruit, vegetables, whole grains, milk, and yogurt are naturally very low in sodium! These lower fat carb choices are loaded with potassium and magnesium. Additionally, fat free milk and fat free yogurt are excellent sources of calcium. Collectively, these nutrients improve artery healthy and help reverse high blood pressure. There's more. Lower fat carbs such as fruit, vegetables, and whole grains are loaded with fiber, yet another essential ingredient in the fight against reversing high blood pressure. All six food strategies in section four contain high levels of artery healthy nutrients. After all, it's all about the arteries.

Eliminate Carbohydrates-Eliminate Anti-Oxidants

Among the many benefits of traditional lower fat heart healthy diets, perhaps their greatest contribution towards preventing ill states comes from their anti-oxidant status. In the insulin resistant state, your blood is compromised. Free radicals produced by your gluco and fat toxic states are destroying your artery lining and your pancreas. To help fight the radicals, you need anti-radicals known as anti-oxidants. Anti-oxidants work by disarming or neutralizing free radicals rendering them harmless. One of your goals in defeating weight related insulin resistance is to keep your blood levels of anti-oxidants as high as possible. Plant foods such as fruit, vegetables, beans, and whole grains offer a plethora of anti-radicals. One of the strongest arguments in favor of lower fat good carbs is their unmatched ability to offer disease fighting anti-oxidants. Higher protein diets, discussed next, are likely to be extremely low in disease fighting anti-oxidants.

One Additional Feature of Plants

In addition to their plethora of anti-oxidants, vitamins and minerals, fiber, low total and saturated fat content, and high water content, plants offer you *super components* known as phytocompounds or phytonutrients. Phytonutrients are another source of anti-oxidants.

There are several reasons these foods have been included in your food portfolio.
- They provide health benefits beyond basic nutrition
- Small quantities afford you their full protection
- They fight free radicals
- You can only obtain their benefits by eating plants!
- They are not found in food of animal origin

I have listed quite a few phytonutrients in the table. There are many more. In fact, close to 1,000 plant compounds are associated with the prevention and treatment of at least four of the leading causes of death in the United States. Fruit and vegetables are your best source. Following absorption, phytonutrients circulate until they capture free radicals.

To this day, I cannot believe how many adults living with some form of chronic disease such as obesity or weight related insulin resistance or high blood pressure or abnormal cholesterol still believe in restricting or eliminating carbs. Eating lower fat good carbs is not only a proven weight loss strategy it's your sole defense against toxic blood. Isn't it ironic that as children we were constantly reminded to "eat fruit and vegetables", but as adults who are *at least overweight* and living with chronic disease, they are forbidden foods. With all of their disease fighting properties, these are the exact foods that need to be consumed regularly, and especially in the insulin resistant state. Yes, they do convert to sugar, but if you consume them in appropriate portions and space them evenly throughout your day, you will avoid blood glucose surges. If only we were more educated as children and adolescents as to why we should have eaten lower fat good carbs, we wouldn't be facing an escalating prevalence of obesity related disease states.

The average American consumes less than one and a half servings of vegetables and less than one serving of fruit per day. Far less that the nearly one pound of fruit and vegetables recommended by the World Health Organization (WHO) study group on diet, nutrition, and prevention of communicable diseases. When you begin consuming the recommended amounts of lower fat good carbs each day in place of other calories, insulin will once again be in control of nutrient trafficking. And don't forget, as you lose weight eating good carbs, your waist circumference shrinks, which decreases your heart and artery disease risk. If these plant foods are combined with healthy fats and lean proteins, you will be impressed with the results of your next blood work. All of this has been planned for you as you progress through the multiple levels of food strategies in section four. The food strategies are designed to teach you how to incorporate carbs into optimal daily food strategies.

PHYTONUTRIENT TABLE

Food (all Carbs)	Phytonutrient	How It Protects You
Apple	Caffeic, Ferulic acid	Antioxidant
Apricots	Beta-Carotene	Antioxidant
Arugula	Zeaxanthin	Antioxidant
Barley	Phytic acid	Antioxidant
Blackberries	Ellagic acid	Antioxidant
Black Eye Peas	Catechin, Epicatechin	Antioxidant
Black Tea	Catechins	Cancer Inhibitor
Blueberry	Caffeic, Ferulic acid	Antioxidant
Bok Choy	Isothiocyanates	Blocks Carcinogens
Broccoli	Isothiocynates	Blocks Carcinogens
Brussels Sprouts	Sulfaforaphane	Blocks Carcinogens
Cabbage	Isothiocyanates, Indoles	Blocks Carcinogens
Carrots	Beta-carotene	Protects Immune System
Cayenne Pepper	Capsaicin	Anti-inflammatory
Cherry	Caffeic, Ferulic acid	Antioxidant
Cauliflower	Isothiocyanates, Indoles	Blocks Carcinogens
Celery	Apigenin	May slow tumor growth
	Quercetin	Promote prostate health
Chili Pepper	Capsaicin	Anti-inflammatory
Cilantro	Carotenoids	Blocks Carcinogens
Collard greens	Lutein/Zeaxanthin	Antioxidant
Cranberries	Ellagic acid	Antioxidant
Curry	Cumarin	Antioxidant
Dark green plants	Carotenoids	Blocks Carcinogens
Flaxseed	Lignans	Cancer reduction

Food (all Carbs)	Phytonutrient	How It Protects You
Garlic	Allyl Sulfides	Antioxidant
Ginger	Gingerol	Antioxidant
Grapes	Ellagic acid	Antioxidant
	Catechin, Epicatechin	Antioxidant
Grapefruit	Caffeic, Ferulic acid	Antioxidant
Green Tea	Catechin	Blocks Carcinogens
Horseradish	Zeaxanthin	Antioxidant
Kale	Zeaxanthin	Antioxidant
Kiwi	Lycopene	Reduce prostate disease
Lentils	Catechin, Epicatechin	Antioxidant
Oats	Phytic acid	Antioxidant
Onions	Allyl Sulfides	Detoxifies
Orange	Caffeic, Ferulic acid	Antioxidant
Strawberries	Ellagic acid, Elligitanins	Antioxidant
Tomato	Lycopene	Antioxidant
Watermelon	Lycopene	Antioxidant

Issues with Traditional Lower Fat Diets

The main complaint of a lower fat diet if you're suffering with weight related insulin resistance is the possibility of elevated triglycerides.

Elevated Triglycerides Results in Low HDL Cholesterol

If you end up with elevated triglycerides in the insulin resistant state, you're likely to end up with fewer and smaller HDL's. To prevent the hypertriglyceridemic state, you must implement a carbohydrate controlled snack and meal strategy. It doesn't mean you have to eliminate carbs. It means you have to distribute carbohydrate grams evenly throughout the day. By controlling carb quantity, you prevent low blood HDL cholesterol.

In Favor of Traditional Lower Fat Diets

The traditional lower fat diet is one strategy that will work to reverse weight related insulin resistance and co-existing ill states such as high cholesterol and hypertension. It never intended to promote the overindulgence of any type of carb, especially refined, processed, and fat free types. Blaming carbohydrate or carbohydrate aliases such as sucrose (table sugar), high fructose corn syrup, corn sweetener, corn syrup, brown sugar, or fruit juice concentrate isn't totally accurate and only a small part of the evidence against weight related insulin resistance. Weight related insulin resistance results from years of faulty nutrition combined with a lack of regular exercise. The lower fat diet was meant to replace dietary fat and cholesterol calories with equal "good" carb calories. You should reconsider carbohydrates. Take a look at the tables and highlights of all six levels in section four. They provide you with an overview of just how healthy a varied food strategy can be.

25 Lower Carb Diets & Insulin Resistance

While traditional lower fat diets do improve weight related insulin resistant states, lower carb proponents claim the same. Here's a look at the claims.

Lower Carb Diets, Weight Loss, and Insulin Resistance

There is no magic behind higher protein diets when it comes to weight loss. If you're looking for the answer as to why high protein diets result in rapid weight loss, look no further than fewer calories consumed, plain and simple. Greater intakes of dietary protein promote greater satiety or "fullness" as protein takes longer to digest. The longer it takes to digest and metabolize, the longer you remain full and the less you eat! If there was something magical about the way they worked, we would all be consuming more dietary protein, losing weight, and not suffering from diseases such as weight related insulin resistance.

In the short term, lower carb diets do prove to be slightly more effective in promoting weight loss compared to traditional lower fat diets. But, at the end of one year, lower carb diets are not any more significant at keeping the pounds off compared to other diets, including traditional lower fat food strategies.

Lower Carb Diets and Improved Hyperglycemia

It has been proposed that "all carbs are not created equal", especially if your insulin resistant and suffer from hyperglycemia. This brings us to the glycemic index (GI), a tool used to rank carbs based on their ability to raise blood glucose.

The GI system divides carbs into low, medium, and high glycemic categories by assigning them a number. Carbohydrates assigned a score of 70 or more are considered to be high glycemic carbs, which will raise your blood glucose more rapidly compared to a carb with a GI score of 55, a low glycemic food. For example, watermelon has been given a score of 72 versus an apple of the same portion that ranks 55. The watermelon would be considered the "high" glycemic fruit, while the apple would be considered the "low" glycemic fruit. Lower glycemic carbs are the better choice compared to higher glycemic carbs as they have a less dramatic impact on existing hyperglycemia.

Food Combining

One way to negate the effects of a high glycemic carb is to food combine. When carbs, regardless of their GI ranking, are combined with protein and or fat, the blood glucose response is blunted. For example, white bread is considered a high glycemic carb. If consumed alone, blood glucose would spike. But, if you add cheese or turkey (protein) to the bread, the sugar from the carb is absorbed much slower as it competes with protein for entry into the blood. This results in a minimal glucose surge.

The Glycemic Index Long Term

The glycemic index is a tool that promotes lower blood glucose. Unfortunately, in the long run when blood glucose management matters most, eliminating a food based on its ability to raise blood glucose by itself is unrealistic. Typically, a food nutrient such as carbohydrate is combined with fat and or protein, thus changing the net effect the carb has on your blood glucose. The appropriate food strategy against weight related insulin resistant states doesn't omit carbs. Of course you won't find soda, donuts, or bagels listed in section four. You will find portion controlled carbs combined with protein and or fat distributed evenly throughout your day to prevent blood glucose spikes.

Lower Carb Diets and Improved Blood Triglycerides

Lower carb diets will improve high blood triglycerides. By eating fewer total carbs, less glucose enters your liver. This results in fewer glucose converted triglycerides that are eventually shipped into the blood.

Lower Carb Diets and Improved HDL Cholesterol

With decreased carb consumption fewer triglyceride transporters (VLDL's) will be released from your liver. With less released into the blood, HDL's hold onto their cholesterol. This keeps them larger in size and therefore cardio protective as they are less likely to be removed by your liver.

Lower Carb Diets and Improved LDL Cholesterol

Sheer weight loss resulting from consuming fewer total calories following a lower carb diet is responsible for lowering blood LDL cholesterol. Any calorie restricted diet that produces weight loss will produce lower LDL cholesterol. Protein rich diets provide no magic in LDL lowering. As much as a 60% reduction in LDL cholesterol may occur when weight loss is achieved.

Issues with Lower Carb Diets

Lower carb diets are relatively "new". The long term effects of these diets on weight and weight related insulin resistance are yet to be determined as the majority of research has been of very short duration. There are several issues that remain quite controversial with lower carb diets.

First, higher protein diets are boring. They offer fewer food choices compared to lower fat diets. Boring diets just aren't as interesting to your appetite. As a result, fewer calories are consumed. However, when appetite does return and it always will, so do calories and eventually body weight.

Second, low carb diets cannot guarantee weight loss. If you replace equal portions of carbs with protein calories you may gain weight.

Third, a higher protein diet is likely to be higher in total and saturated fat and dietary cholesterol. While some dietary fat is needed, saturated fat and dietary cholesterol are toxic to your insulin resistant state. You can't afford any more damage to your arteries, liver, muscles, or pancreas.

Fourth, lower carb diets are likely to be higher in sodium, which will exacerbate existing hypertension.

26 Supplements & Insulin Resistance

Since food is the primary link between the overweight state and heart and artery disease, food should be used to reverse your overweight state, not supplements. When it comes to protecting your cells, pills simply cannot do the work of food nutrients. Food as a whole (food synergy) is responsible for your long-term health. Too many people are caught up in believing that mega dosing a single nutrient supplement will reverse what years of faulty nutrition has created. Regardless of how strong the supplement claims are, they are band-aids. Some supplements treat symptoms, but none teach or motivate you to make habit forming lifestyle changes. If you researched it enough, you would find that just about every supplement out there would have a positive impact on treating weight related insulin resistant states. No single pill, drink, or powder has ever reversed the disease promoting effects of excess body weight.

About Supplements

If you are thinking of using a synthetic form of nutrition, there are a few questions you should pursue before purchasing the supplement.

1. Is the supplement pure?
2. Do you know what the ingredients are?

3. Are the ingredients obtainable from food?
4. Does the supplement metabolize as food nutrients do?
5. Many supplements contain mega doses of nutrients. Is this safe?
6. Are there side effects?

Research the supplement, ask questions, and look at credible studies done on the product rather than the manufacturers website. Did you know that only 10-15% of a multivitamin/mineral supplement is used by your body while a much greater percentage of fiber and nutrients such as folate, vitamin C, potassium, magnesium, vitamin A, vitamin E, selenium, and zinc can be absorbed and used from foods?

The Irony Behind Supplements

Isn't it ironic that vitamins and minerals are required in milligrams or micrograms (extremely small quantities), yet we think mega dosing massive quantities is healthier for us? Isn't it ironic that we spend tens of billions of dollars a year on synthetic nutrients that can be obtained from high quality, fiber, and vitamin and mineral rich relatively inexpensive foods? It's ironic that many of our synthetic forms of nutrition are nearly calorie free, yet we are the world's most overweight and obese society. You need calories to lose body fat! It's crazy if you think about it, but more than 50% of adults use supplements regularly to manage their health, yet more than 60% of adults are at least overweight.

The Truth Behind Supplements

The claims made for or against synthetic nutrition are always changing. New conclusions are always being drawn that may not be in support of what was once thought to be established. On the contrary, the claims in favor of fruit, vegetables, and other whole intact grains have only strengthened, especially when it comes to fighting weight related insulin resistant states.

You need to understand there are side effects of healthy food strategies in the insulin resistant state. They include weight loss and maintenance, improved insulin sensitivity, lower fasting blood glucose, improved blood cholesterol, lower blood pressure, and lower blood triglycerides. Perhaps most important, regular exercise and the proper daily food strategies are your only true means of long term prevention. Don't be naïve or fooled into what ads, magazines, and commercials are trying to promote. They are not always looking out for your best interest. Eat food!

SECTION IV

THE FOOD STRATEGIES

27 Weight Related Insulin Resistant Food Strategies

If 3,500 calories equal one pound, gained or lost, then a calorie is a calorie, regardless of the source. If you create a caloric deficit by consuming fewer calories, by exercising, or by consuming fewer calories combined with exercise, you begin "freeing up" space in your fat cells. This allows them to function more efficiently. If they function as they should, your cells become more tolerant to glucose and more sensitive to insulin. In other words, glucose doesn't get stuck outside your cells causing a back up of glucose. Simply stated, weight loss and weight maintenance is the absolute best way to improve insulin's rule over carbohydrate and fat metabolism. So, the answer to the sixty four thousand dollar question "*is there an optimal diet prescription to treat weight related insulin resistant states is a big fat no*". Any "diet" that helps you stay focused on losing and then maintaining body weight will improve insulin resistance and the conditions that so often accompany it. Here's the best news. The composition of your diet, as in the percentage of carb, protein, or fat doesn't matter either. It's your call as it ultimately boils down to calories. Lower fat or lower carb diets both produce very similar results. Don't be enticed by how quickly others have lost weight or how fast a "plan" claims to work. It took years to earn your unwanted waist circumference. Don't be in a hurry to reverse the conditions it has caused as it will lead to greater suffering. There are no magic bullets, quick fixes, short cuts, gimmicks, or pills, only food strategies.

The Food Strategies

Now that you know there is no special or optimal diet to treat any weight related chronic disease, you do need to understand there are food nutrients and food strategies that will give you the tools to reverse and control weight related insulin resistance.

In all, there are six progressive levels. Start with level one as forming habits will be a key factor to your success.

Levels one and two are simple snacking options. They provide you with solutions to common day to day issues regarding what to eat between meals. Weight loss is not intended with either level. Level three is a continuation of level two. It comes packed with the appropriate chronic disease fighting snacks, plus it begins providing food suggestions at meals. Levels four, five, and six are complete weight related insulin resistant food strategies. Don't forget to look at the tables and read the highlights of each level. You're going to be very motivated.

How Much Weight Should You Expect to Lose?

Beginning at level four, women should start at the 1,200-1,300 calorie plan, which is the strategy listed. Men should start with the 1,500 calorie plan. This is the plan listed plus the additional food portions under the 1,500 calorie column.

Since everyone is different, it's difficult to precisely tell you how many pounds of fat you should lose each day, each week, or month. There are an exceptional number of variables that affect weight loss. They include starting body weight, fat to muscle ratio, age, gender, exercise, metabolism, and commitment to behavior change.

In general, a healthy and sustainable weight loss of up to two pounds a week can be expected. As your body undergoes chemical and metabolic changes, your weight loss will vary week to week. Don't be discouraged if one week you lose two pounds and the next week only a half. Fat loss should be measured over 30, 60, and 90 days, not over a single week. Be patient.

If you are losing weight each week, stay with your current plan. If you are losing more than 2 pounds per week, most weeks, the plan is overly restrictive. If this is the case, move up one hundred calories per day. For example, if you are losing more than two pounds per week on the 1,200-1,300 calorie plan, begin following the 1,400 calorie plan. This should slow the rate of weight loss to a more sustainable pace. Give it a few weeks to slow. If you are still losing more than two pounds after two weeks, increase your intake another hundred calories. Don't be tricked into thinking a rapid weight loss is healthy, it's not! It's unrealistic, too restrictive, and sets you up for weight regain.

After you finish with level six, you will have the tools to manage weight related insulin resistant states. More important, you will have established optimal eating habits! If your latest blood work shows signs of improved glucose tolerance, insulin sensitivity, blood cholesterol and triglycerides, and lower blood pressure, congratulations, maintain your current course! If you feel further improvements are needed or are looking to stay on track, consider these exercise components. If you implement one or more of these variables, you're going to add calories.

Duration

Duration or how long you exercise will boost your metabolism resulting in more calories burned and eventually weight loss. If you exercise for an hour a day, begin increasing your exercise time by 25% or 15 additional minutes per workout. While it doesn't seem like much, it ends up being one extra hour per week.

Frequency

By increasing how often you exercise or the frequency of your workouts, expect weight related benefits. Start by adding half of the exercise you normally do on one of your days off. Do this for several weeks before turning the half workout into a full session.

Intensity

Once you have maximized the duration and frequency, consider increasing the intensity of your workout. Start by making one of your workouts more rigorous. This can be achieved by adding more repetitions or heavier weight or both to a single workout. If you run on a treadmill, change the intensity by increasing the speed or the grade to a higher incline or both. You will only have to increase the intensity for part of your workout as it will take a toll on your energy levels rather quickly. If you enjoy walking outside, intensity can be increased by walking up hill or by fast walking or even jogging for very short intervals. Intense workouts are excellent for energizing you and shocking your system.

They burn more calories but are risky in terms of injury, so one per week or four per month to begin with is plenty.

How Many Calories Should I Add?

Begin by adding 100 to 200 calories extra per day for as long as you change one or more of the variables.

Exercise Benefits of Weight Related Insulin Resistance

While it sounds a bit odd, you're going to continue to lose weight by adding extra calories each day. The more you exercise the more muscle you build. This results in a more efficient fat burning process. Fat burning also occurs at rest as muscle mass always has to be fed! This sequence of events directly improves insulin resistance!

Specifically, you should expect improved blood pressure. As you lose weight, blood pressure will decrease as it's directly proportional to your body weight. Lower blood triglycerides and low density lipoprotein (LDL) cholesterol will also result as will improvements in overall cell efficiency. Your fasting blood glucose will improve significantly as your liver and working muscles become much more efficient at metabolizing glucose. In fact, exercise of any type allows your muscles to open up with insulin stimulation! Imagine how relieved your arteries will be. You pancreas will greatly appreciate your exercise efforts as it will be able to rest more and work less.

Level 1 Weight Related Insulin Resistant Food Strategy

Level one is your starting point. It's a snacking strategy that's meant to be a building block in the fight against weight related insulin resistant states. Snacks can be thought of as smaller meals. Smaller quantities of calories spread throughout the day help control cravings and prevent overeating at meals. Snacking is an excellent way to begin learning portion control. If you eat smaller amounts of food you will lose weight. Weight loss improves all insulin resistant states. Snacking also provides your body with vitamin and mineral rich "good" calories that help support your immune system.

What About Your Meals?

What you eat at breakfast, lunch, and dinner is up to you right now. Keep in mind you will be snacking after breakfast and after lunch, so give up several bites of whatever you're eating at those meals to save room for my snack suggestions. Level one is not intended to be a complete chronic disease fighting food strategy. Instead, it's a habit forming strategy. *Start by snacking on carbohydrate controlled foods that provide nearly the same number of calories and total carbohydrate grams at each snack. This essential step will help prevent large fluctuations in blood glucose.*

AVERAGES

	Calories	Carbohydrate (g)
Snack 1	107	14
Snack 2	113	11

LEVEL 1 RECOMMENDATIONS

1. Snack one should come somewhere between breakfast and lunch. It is best to have snack two approximately two hours before dinner as it will help prevent overeating at dinner. If you choose to eat snack two after dinner, wait two hours.
2. You should not skip breakfast regardless of when you begin your day. Skipping breakfast will result in higher fasting blood glucose and the likelihood of overeating later in the day. Do not use snack one in place of breakfast.
3. You should not skip meals. Level one is intended to provide you with snacks in addition to meals. If you normally skip or avoid meals, begin providing your body with calories from food at breakfast, lunch, and dinner. Calorie inconsistency is one reason you suffer from abnormal glucose metabolism.
4. You should not skip snacks. If you are not hungry at a recommended snack time, eat half of the snack. Calories support energy, provide adequate and continuous nutrients, and prevent overeating at meals.
5. All snack strategies are interchangeable. You may eat snack two first.
6. Water is encouraged. Since everyone is different, water needs are different. Exercise, temperature, humidity, and food choices make a difference in the amount of water used and therefore needed. General recommendations are to consume between 3 and 4 liters of water per day. Drinking water while snacking is an excellent way to achieve water recommendations.
7. If you consume diet drinks, coffee, or any type of beverage made with a sugar substitute, you need to be very careful. They are mild diuretics, which may increase water loss, lead to slight dehydration, and stimulate overeating as a result of their sweet taste.
8. Portion control is crucial. I would recommend that you purchase a very inexpensive set of measuring cups to help teach you the serving sizes listed.

SUBSTITUTION LIST

Below is a list of interchangeable foods. You can substitute foods listed in any food strategy with the foods below, just be sure to follow the portion sizes listed. Substituting may alter averages and compositions slightly.

Berries	Blue, Straw, Rasp, Black
Butter	Peanut, Almond, Cashew
Fish*	Halibut, Haddock, Orange Roughy
Hummus	Regular, Flavored
Milk	Non-fat, Soy, Almond, Low-fat Lactaid
Nuts	Almonds, Walnuts, Peanuts, Pistachios
Oil	Olive, Canola, Rice Bran
Potatoes	Yam, Sweet
Spreads	Smart Balance®, Benecol Light®, Promise Activ®

* where salmon is listed, do not substitute

Level 1

Day 1

Snack 1 — 5-6 apple slices, with skin + 2 tablespoons sliced/slivered almonds, unsalted
102 Calories, 10 grams total Carbohydrate

Snack 2 — 2 cups lite microwave popcorn or 2 cups air popped popcorn + 2 tablespoons almonds, unsalted
167 Calories, 16 grams total Carbohydrate
Or-
6" whole-wheat tortilla + 1 tablespoon reduced fat peanut butter
154 Calories, 7 grams total Carbohydrate

Day 2

Snack 1 — 1/3 cup of any whole grain cereal, with 5 or more grams of fiber per serving + 2 tablespoons sliced or slivered almonds, unsalted
120 Calories, 16 grams total Carbohydrate

Snack 2 — 5-6 apple slices + 1/3 cup non-fat or low-fat cottage cheese
79 Calories, 10 grams total Carbohydrate
Or-
6" whole-wheat tortilla + 1 tablespoon reduced fat peanut butter
154 Calories, 25 grams total Carbohydrate

Day 3

Snack 1 — 1 cup diced cantaloupe + 4 walnut halves
110 Calories, 15 grams total Carbohydrate

Snack 2 — ½ cup soybeans (edamame), boiled, unsalted
127 Calories, 10 grams total Carbohydrate
Or-
1 medium orange + 2 tablespoons sliced or slivered almonds, unsalted
133 Calories, 18 grams total Carbohydrate

Day 4
Snack 1 — 3 oz low-fat or non-fat yogurt, plain or fruit flavored + 2 tablespoons crushed walnuts
95 Calories, 9 grams total Carbohydrate

Snack 2 — 4 small whole-wheat crackers + 1 tablespoon reduced fat peanut butter
152 Calories, 15 grams total Carbohydrate
Or-
5-6 baby carrots + 1 tablespoon reduced fat peanut butter
110 Calories, 8 grams total Carbohydrate

Day 5
Snack 1 — 1/3 cup whole grain cereal with 5 or more grams fiber per serving, dry + 2 tablespoons sliced almonds, unsalted
120 Calories, 16 grams total Carbohydrate

Snack 2 — 1 cup honeydew + 1/3 cup low-fat or non-fat cottage cheese
108 Calories, 18 grams total Carbohydrate
Or-
½ cup soybeans (edamame), boiled, no salt
127 Calories, 10 grams total Carbohydrate

Day 6
Snack 1 — 1/3 cup low-fat or non-fat cottage cheese + ½ cup sliced strawberries, fresh or frozen
73 Calories, 8 grams total Carbohydrate

Snack 2 — 3 oz tuna, canned in water, drained, roll into lettuce leaf, have 2
103 Calories, 1 gram total Carbohydrate
Or-
4 whole-wheat crackers + 3 oz tuna, in water, drained
170 Calories, 11 grams total Carbohydrate

Day 7

Snack 1 — ½ cup blueberries, fresh or frozen + 1/3 cup non-fat or low-fat cottage cheese
88 Calories, 12 grams total Carbohydrate

Snack 2 — Medium orange + 4 walnut halves
113 Calories, 17 grams total Carbohydrate
Or-
5-6 baby carrots + 1 tablespoon reduced fat peanut butter
110 Calories, 9 grams total Carbohydrate

Day 8

Snack 1 — 1 cup honeydew or cantaloupe, diced + 4 walnut halves
111 Calories, 17 grams total Carbohydrate

Snack 2 — 1/3 cup whole grain cereal with 5 or more grams fiber per serving, dry + 2 tablespoons sliced almonds, unsalted
120 Calories, 16 grams total Carbohydrate
Or-
½ cup soybeans (edamame), boiled, no salt
127 Calories, 10 grams total Carbohydrate

Day 9

Snack 1 — 1/3 cup non-fat or low-fat yogurt, plain or fruit flavored + 2 tablespoons sliced/slivered almonds, unsalted
114 Calories, 9 grams total Carbohydrate

Snack 2 — ½ cup sliced strawberries, fresh + 6 almonds, dry roasted, unsalted
106 Calories, 10 grams total Carbohydrate
Or-
2 cups air popped popcorn or 2 cups lite microwave popcorn + 4 walnut halves
113 Calories, 14 grams total Carbohydrate

Day 10

Snack 1 1/3 cup whole grain cereal, with 5 or more grams fiber per serving, dry + 2 tablespoons sliced/slivered almonds, unsalted
120 Calories, 16 grams total Carbohydrate

Snack 2 ½ cup soybeans (edamame), boiled, no salt
127 Calories, 10 grams total Carbohydrate
Or-
5-6 apple slices + 1 reduced fat string cheese (1 oz)
110 Calories, 9 grams total Carbohydrate

Day 11

Snack 1 ½ cup sliced strawberries, fresh + 1/3 cup non-fat or low-fat cottage cheese
73 Calories, 8 grams total Carbohydrate

Snack 2 1 cup honeydew or cantaloupe, diced + 6 almonds, unsalted
166 Calories, 19 grams total Carbohydrate
Or-
Medium celery stalk (6-7"), cut into pieces + 1 tablespoon reduced fat peanut butter
90 Calories, 8 grams total Carbohydrate

Day 12

Snack 1 ¼ cup low-fat cottage cheese + 1.5 cups honeydew or cantaloupe
114 Calories, 16 grams total Carbohydrate

Snack 2 ½ cup blueberries, fresh or frozen + 4 walnut halves
92 Calories, 12 grams total Carbohydrate
Or-
3 oz tuna, canned in water, drained, roll into lettuce leaf, have 2
103 Calories, 1 gram total Carbohydrate

Day 13
Snack 1   Whole-wheat tortilla (6") + 1 tablespoon reduced fat peanut butter
154 Calories, 25 grams total Carbohydrate

Snack 2   5-6 baby carrots mixed with 5-6 red pepper slices + 2 tablespoons lite Italian dressing
52 Calories, 6 grams total Carbohydrate
Or-
½ cup soybeans (edamame), boiled, no salt
127 Calories, 10 grams total Carbohydrate

Day 14
Snack 1   5-6 apple slices + 1 tablespoon reduced fat peanut butter
102 Calories, 10 grams total Carbohydrate

Snack 2   ½ cup sliced strawberries, fresh or frozen + 1/3 cup non-fat or low-fat cottage cheese
73 Calories, 8 grams total Carbohydrate
Or-
5-6 baby carrots mixed with 5-6 red pepper slices + 2 tablespoons lite Italian dressing
52 Calories, 17 grams total Carbohydrate

Congratulations. Habits are the key to your success. Here are your next 14 days.

Level 2 Weight Related Insulin Resistant Food Strategy

Level two provides you with <u>one</u> additional calorie and carb controlled snack. Snacks are recommended before lunch, before dinner, and after dinner. *The objective of level two is to provide you with vitamin and mineral rich snacks that are spaced evenly throughout the day.* It's not intended to be a complete chronic disease fighting food strategy. Rather, it builds on your current habit of snacking to fight weight related insulin resistance. Benefits of level two include minimizing saturated fat and therefore total fat calories. Keeping saturated fat to a minimum helps metabolize glucose. Snacks are even controlled for sodium. Many who are insulin resistant suffer from elevated blood pressure or hypertension. Low sodium and sodium free snack foods are used to help prevent further abnormalities in blood pressure. Additionally, all 14 snacks are rich in dietary fiber, which promotes fullness, prevents overeating, reduces blood sugar surges, and helps control blood pressure!

What About Your Meals?

What you eat at breakfast, lunch, and dinner, is up to you right now. You will be snacking before lunch, before dinner, and after dinner. With that in mind, give up a few bites of whatever you're eating at meals.

AVERAGES

	Calories	Carbs (g)	Total Fat (g)	Sat Fat (g)	Sodium (mg)	Fiber (g)
Snack 1	104	12	4.7	<1	117	2.9
Snack 2	115	12	5.5	<1	118	2.8
Snack 3	90	7	4.4	1	103	1.6

LEVEL 2 RECOMMENDATIONS

1. You may choose to have snack three as a second afternoon snack before dinner. If you choose to do this, be sure to allow approximately two hours after lunch. For example, if you eat your lunch at 1 pm, then snack two should be at or close to 3 pm followed by snack three at or around 5 pm. Dinner would follow at or close to 7 pm.
2. You should not skip breakfast regardless of when you begin your day. Skipping breakfast will result in higher fasting blood glucose and the likelihood of overeating later in the day. Do not use snack one in place of breakfast.
3. You should not skip meals. Level two is intended to provide you with snacks in addition to meals. Snacking promotes fullness and helps maintain calorie and carb consistency throughout the day. If you normally skip meals, begin providing your body with calories from food at breakfast, lunch, and dinner. Calorie inconsistency is one reason you suffer from abnormal glucose metabolism.
4. You should not skip snacks. If you are not hungry at a recommended snack time, eat half of the snack. Calories support energy, provide adequate and continuous nutrients, and prevent overeating at meals.
5. All snack strategies are interchangeable.
6. Water is encouraged. Since everyone is different, water needs are different. Exercise, temperature, humidity, and food choices make a difference in the amount of water used and therefore needed. General recommendations are to consume between 3 and 4 liters of water per day. Drinking water while snacking is an excellent way to achieve water recommendations.
7. If you consume diet drinks, coffee, or any type of beverage made with a sugar substitute, you need to be very careful. They are mild diuretics, which may increase water loss, lead to slight dehydration, and stimulate over eating as a result of their sweet taste.
8. Portion control is crucial. I would recommend purchasing a very inexpensive set of measuring cups to help teach you the serving sizes listed.

Level 2

Day 1

Snack 1   5-6 apple slices, with skin + 2 tablespoons sliced or slivered almonds, unsalted

Snack 2   2 cups air popped popcorn + 2 tablespoons almonds, dry roasted, unsalted
Or-
6" whole-wheat tortilla + 1 tablespoon peanut butter

Snack 3   Medium celery stalk (6-7"), cut into pieces + 1 tablespoon peanut butter

	Calories	Carbs (g)	Total Fat (g)	Sat Fat (g)	Sodium (mg)	Fiber (g)
Snack 1	102	10	6	<1	0	2
Snack 2	167	15.3	10	1	1.1	4.4
Or-						
Snack 2	118	15	5.2	1	175	2
Snack 3	91	7.4	5.3	1	151	2

Day 2

Snack 1 — 1/3 cup of any whole grain cereal, with 5 or more grams of fiber per serving + 2 tablespoons sliced or slivered almonds, unsalted

Snack 2 — 5-6 apple slices + 1/3 cup non-fat or low-fat cottage cheese
Or-
6" whole-wheat tortilla + 1 tablespoon peanut butter

Snack 3 — 6 almonds, dry roasted, unsalted

	Calories	Carbs (g)	Total Fat (g)	Sat Fat (g)	Sodium (mg)	Fiber (g)
Snack 1	121	16	6.5	<1	38	7.2
Snack 2	79	10	1	<1	228	1
Or-						
Snack 2	118	15	5.2	1	175	2
Snack 3	122	3	9	<1	.5	2

Day 3

Snack 1	1 cup diced cantaloupe + 4 walnut halves, unsalted
Snack 2	½ cup soybeans (edamame), boiled, unsalted Or- 1 medium orange + 2 tablespoons sliced or slivered almonds, unsalted
Snack 3	Low sodium cheese (1 oz)

	Calories	Carbs (g)	Total Fat (g)	Sat Fat (g)	Sodium (mg)	Fiber (g)
Snack 1	110	14.5	5.5	<1	15	1.5
Snack 2	127	10	6	<1	13	4
Or-						
Snack 2	132	18	6	<1	0	4
Snack 3	79	1	5	3	4.5	0

Day 4

Snack 1   3 oz low-fat or non-fat yogurt, plain or fruit flavored + 2 tablespoons crushed walnuts, unsalted

Snack 2   4 small whole-wheat crackers (2" x 2") + 1 tablespoon peanut butter
Or-
5-6 baby carrots + 1 tablespoon peanut butter

Snack 3   1/3 cup low-fat or non-fat cottage cheese + ½ cup sliced strawberries, fresh or frozen

	Calories	Carbs (g)	Total Fat (g)	Sat Fat (g)	Sodium (mg)	Fiber (g)
Snack 1	95	8.5	5	<1	51	.8
Snack 2	152	15	8	1.5	193	2.5
Or-						
Snack 2	110	9	5.8	1	106	1.9
Snack 3	73	8	1.2	<1	229	2

Day 5

Snack 1	1/3 cup whole grain cereal with 5 or more grams fiber per serving, dry + 2 tablespoons sliced or slivered almonds, unsalted
Snack 2	1 cup honeydew + 1/3 cup low-fat or non-fat cottage cheese Or- ½ cup soybeans (edamame), boiled, no salt
Snack 3	2 cups air popped popcorn + 1 tablespoon grated parmesan cheese, sprinkled

	Calories	Carbs (g)	Total Fat (g)	Sat Fat (g)	Sodium (mg)	Fiber (g)
Snack 1	120	16	6.5	<1	38	7.2
Snack 2	108	18	1	<1	245	1
Or-						
Snack 2	127	10	6	<1	13	4.8
Snack 3	89	12.25	2.4	1.2	117	2.4

Day 6

Snack 1	1/3 cup low-fat or non-fat cottage cheese + ½ cup sliced strawberries, fresh or frozen
Snack 2	3 oz tuna, canned in water, drained, roll into lettuce leaf, have 2 Or- 4 whole-wheat crackers (2"x 2") + 3 oz tuna, in water, drained
Snack 3	Medium celery stalk (6-7"), cut into pieces + 1 tablespoon peanut butter

	Calories	Carbs (g)	Total Fat (g)	Sat Fat (g)	Sodium (mg)	Fiber (g)
Snack 1	73	8	1.2	<1	229	2
Snack 2	103	1	.7	0	289	.3
Or-						
Snack 2	170	11	1.1	<1	392	1.6
Snack 3	90	8	5.7	1	140	2

Day 7

Snack 1   ½ cup blueberries, fresh or frozen + 1/3 cup non-fat or low-fat cottage cheese

Snack 2   medium orange + 4 walnut halves, unsalted
Or-
5-6 baby carrots + 1 tablespoon peanut butter

Snack 3   6 almonds or 4 walnut halves, dry roasted, unsalted

	Calories	Carbs (g)	Total Fat (g)	Sat Fat (g)	Sodium (mg)	Fiber (g)
Snack 1	88	12	1.2	<1	233	2
Snack 2	113	16.5	5	<1	1	3.3
Or-						
Snack 2	110	9	5.8	1	106	1.9
Snack 3	106	3.3	9	1	.5	2

Day 8

Snack 1   1 cup honeydew or cantaloupe, diced + 4 walnut halves, unsalted

Snack 2   1/3 cup whole grain cereal with 5 or more grams fiber per serving, dry + 2 tablespoons sliced almonds, unsalted
Or-
½ cup soybeans (edamame), boiled, no salt

Snack 3   3-4 apple slices + low sodium cheese (1 oz)

	Calories	Carbs (g)	Total Fat (g)	Sat Fat (g)	Sodium (mg)	Fiber (g)
Snack1	111	16.5	5.25	<1	18	1.3
Snack 2	120	16	6.5	<1	38	7.2
Or-						
Snack 2	127	10	6	<1	13	4.8
Snack 3	110	9	5.25	3	5	1

Day 9

Snack 1 — 1/3 cup non-fat or low-fat yogurt, plain or fruit flavored + 2 tablespoons sliced or slivered almonds, unsalted

Snack 2 — ½ cup sliced strawberries, fresh or frozen + 6 almonds, dry roasted, unsalted
Or-
2 cups air popped popcorn or 2 cups lite microwave popcorn + 4 walnut halves, unsalted

Snack 3 — ½ cup sliced strawberries, fresh or frozen + 1/3 cup non-fat or low-fat cottage cheese

	Calories	Carbs (g)	Total Fat (g)	Sat Fat (g)	Sodium (mg)	Fiber (g)
Snack1	114	9	6	<1	50	1.75
Snack 2	106	10	10	<1	1.3	4
Or-						
Snack 2	113	13.5	5.6	<1	1.4	2.6
Snack 3	73	8	1.2	<1	229	2

Day 10

Snack 1 — 1/3 cup whole grain cereal, with 5 or more grams fiber per serving, dry + 2 tablespoons sliced or slivered almonds, unsalted

Snack 2 — ½ cup soybeans (edamame), boiled, no salt
Or-
3-4 apple slices + low sodium cheese (1 oz)

Snack 3 — 2 cups air popped popcorn + 1 tablespoon grated parmesan cheese, sprinkled

	Calories	Carbs (g)	Total Fat (g)	Sat Fat (g)	Sodium (mg)	Fiber (g)
Snack 1	120	16	6.5	<1	38	7.2
Snack 2	127	10	6	<1	13	4.8
Or-						
Snack 2	110	9	5.25	3	5	1
Snack 3	90	12.25	2.6	1.2	117	2.4

Day 11

Snack 1 ½ cup sliced strawberries, fresh or frozen + 1/3 cup non-fat or low-fat cottage cheese

Snack 2 1 medium orange + 2 tablespoons sliced or slivered almonds, unsalted
Or-
Medium celery stalk (6-7"), cut into pieces + 1 tablespoon peanut butter

Snack 3 5-6 red pepper slices + 5-6 cucumber slices + 2 tablespoons lite Italian dressing

	Calories	Carbs (g)	Total Fat (g)	Sat Fat (g)	Sodium (mg)	Fiber (g)
Snack1	73	8	1.2	<1	229	2
Snack 2	132	18	6	<1	0	4
Or-						
Snack 2	90	8	5.7	1	140	2
Snack 3	37	3	3	<1	87	.4

Day 12

Snack 1   ½ cup blueberries, fresh or frozen + 1/3 cup non-fat or low-fat cottage cheese

Snack 2   ½ cup blueberries, fresh or frozen + 4 walnut halves, unsalted
Or-
3 oz tuna, canned in water, drained, roll into 2 loose leaf lettuce pieces

Snack 3   ½ cup blueberries, fresh or frozen + 1 tablespoon peanut butter

	Calories	Carbs (g)	Total Fat (g)	Sat Fat (g)	Sodium (mg)	Fiber (g)
Snack 1	88	12	1.2	<1	233	2
Snack 2	92	11.5	5.5	<1	1.6	2.3
Or-						
Snack 2	103	1	.70	<1	289	.3
Snack 3	121	15	6	1	92	3

Day 13

Snack 1   6" whole-wheat tortilla + 1 tablespoon peanut butter

Snack 2   5-6 baby carrots mixed with 5-6 red pepper slices + 2 tablespoons lite Italian dressing
Or-
½ cup soybeans (edamame), boiled, no salt

Snack 3   6 almonds or 4 walnut halves, dry roasted, unsalted

	Calories	Carbs (g)	Total Fat (g)	Sat Fat (g)	Sodium (mg)	Fiber (g)
Snack1	154	25	5.75	1	260	2.8
Snack 2	52	6	3.2	<1	254	1
Or-						
Snack 2	127	10	6	<1	13	4.8
Snack 3	52	1.5	5	<1	1	.3

Day 14

Snack 1   5-6 apple slices, with skin + 2 tablespoons sliced or slivered almonds, unsalted

Snack 2   ½ cup sliced strawberries, fresh or frozen + 1/3 cup non-fat or low-fat cottage cheese
Or-
5-6 baby carrots mixed with 5-6 red pepper slices + 2 tablespoons lite Italian dressing

Snack 3   1 orange + 2 tablespoon sliced or slivered almonds, unsalted

	Calories	Carbs (g)	Total Fat (g)	Sat Fat (g)	Sodium (mg)	Fiber (g)
Snack1	102	10	6	<1	0	2
Snack 2	73	8	1.2	<1	229	2
Or-						
Snack 2	52	6	3.2	<1	254	1
Snack 3	132	17	5.2	<1	0	4.2

Congratulations on making it 30 days!

Consistency is your key. Snacks have become a regular part of your daily routine. Your body is used to handling smaller amounts of calories. You're earning a smaller waist circumference. Carbohydrate calories are controlled. This results in fewer hunger cues and blood glucose spikes. Welcome aboard.

Level 3 Weight Related Insulin Resistant Food Strategy

You have completed one month of weight related insulin resistant food strategies. Your improvements include, the number of times you eat (eating frequency), the amount of food you eat (quantity), and the quality of your food choices. For example, eating smaller meals more often results in a much more efficient metabolism. This benefits not only your stomach and your waistline, but your blood glucose, blood cholesterol and triglycerides, and blood pressure as well. Food quality coupled with weight loss results in lower blood pressure and improved artery health. Let's not forget all of the vitamins, minerals, anti-oxidants, and plant nutrients that provide synergistic cell health. All of these small changes are the building blocks of the "optimal" weight loss and cardiovascular disease prevention food strategy. Nicely done!

Level three is a continuation of level two. It maintains the snacking and habit forming approach. The addition is partial meal suggestions. You should eat the food listed at each meal plus food from your food portfolio. How much you eat is up to you for now. Eat until you are satisfied. You will begin monitoring the portion size very soon. Where your strategy lists **C**, choose a food that has a (c) next to it. Where your strategy lists **P**, choose a food that has a (p) next to it, and where the strategy lists **F**, choose a food with (f) next to it.

The first new feature of this food strategy includes controlling for carbohydrate quantity and quality. Both are essential "ingredients" in managing and improving weight related insulin resistance. The second feature helps you control your sodium intake. The majority of Americans, not just those who are overweight or obese, have trouble keeping dietary sodium levels within a healthy range. Over time, this takes a toll on your arteries.

Carbohydrate quantity is perhaps the most important aspect of managing elevated blood glucose. Since all carbohydrates digest into glucose, a key to preventing blood glucose surges and therefore hyperglycemia is to control the total amount of carb you consume.

Carbohydrate quality is also important in managing blood glucose. Consuming high quality carbs, those with ample dietary fiber and minimal added sugar help prevent blood glucose "peaks and valleys". All of this has been planned for you here and in the remaining levels.

Don't get caught up in eliminating carbs. It's too unrealistic. It's more important that you learn to exercise portion control of all types of carbs. In all food strategies, the carbohydrate portion of the meal is combined with protein and or fat to prevent blood glucose spikes.

Your take home message regarding carb quantity and quality is this; both matter, but controlling the amount (quantity) ultimately prevents excess blood glucose accumulation and therefore blood insulin concentrations. It's all about portion control!

HIGHLIGHTS

Averages	Meal	Snack
Calories	121	107
Carbohydrate (grams)	19	11
Total Fat (grams)	2.5	5
Saturated Fat (grams)	<1 gram	<1 gram
Fiber (grams)	5	3
Sodium (milligrams)	180	128

Dietary cholesterol kept as close to zero as possible!

If you're curious as to why snacks have more total fat compared to meals, the answer lies in your meals. In most cases, meal times are much higher in total calories and total fat calories. To help balance out inconsistencies between meals and snacks, I have planned fewer fat grams and therefore fewer fat calories at meals. Of course the type of fats I have chosen, the unsaturated ones, the mufas and pufas, will improve insulin resistance and blood lipids. Eat Healthy, Stay Healthy!

FOOD PORTFOLIO
CARBOHYDRATE, PROTEIN, & FAT

Almond butter (f)	Cucumber slices (c)	Pumpkin seeds, unsalted, (f)
Almonds, unsalted (f)	English muffin, whole wheat (c)	Popcorn, lite/air popped (c)
Apple (c)	Flaxseed oil (f)	Quinoa (c)
Asparagus, steamed (c)	Guava (c)	Rice, wild (c)
Avocado (f)	Haddock (p)	Rice, brown (c)
Banana (c)	Halibut (p)	Salmon, canned (p)
Barley (c)	Honeydew (c)	Salmon, wild/farmed (p)
Beans, kidney (c)	Hummus (f)	Sesame seeds (f)
Beans, cannellini (c)	Kiwi (c)	Soybeans (edamame) (c)
Beans, garbanzo (c)	Lentils (c)	Spread, Benecol® (f)
Berries, Blackberries (c)	Low fat cottage cheese (p)	Spread, Benecol Light® (f)
Blueberries (c)	Macadamia nuts (f)	Spinach, raw/steamed (c)
Raspberries (c)	Marinara sauce, low sodium (c)	Squash, summer, baked (c)
Strawberries (c)	Margarine, Smart Balance® (f)	Sunflower seeds, unsalted (f)
Bread, whole wheat (c)	Milk, soy/almond (c)	Tempeh (p)
Bread, rye (c)	Milk, fat free or low fat (c)	Tofu (p)
Broccoli, raw/steam (c)	Mushrooms (c)	Tomatoes (c)
Brussels Sprouts (c)	Oatmeal, instant, plain (c)	Tortilla, whole wheat (c)
Bulgar (c)	Oatmeal, steel cut (c)	Tuna, Starkist, low sod (p)
Brazil nuts (f)	Oats, whole (c)	Chunk white albacore (p)
Canola oil (f)	Okra, fresh/frozen (c)	Turkey, ground/breast (p)
Cantaloupe (c)	Olive oil, extra virgin (f)	T. breast, sliced, low sod (p)
Carrots, baby/shred (c)	Orange (c)	Trout, farmed, wild (p)
Cashews (f)	Pasta, whole wheat (c)	Walnuts (f)
Caulifl. fresh/steam (c)	Peanut butter (f)	Watermelon (c)
Celery (c)	Peanuts, dry roast. unsalted (f)	Whole grain cereal (c)
Chx br. White/n skin (p)	Peppers, red/green/yellow (c)	Whole rye (c)
Chicory (c)	Pistachios (f)	Yam, cooked, mash (c)
Cilantro (c)	Potato, sweet/baked/ mash (c)	Yogurt, plain/flavored
		low or fat free

LEVEL 3 RECOMMENDATIONS

1. You may choose to have snack three as a second afternoon snack before dinner. If you choose to do this, be sure to allow approximately two hours after lunch. For example, if you eat your lunch at 1 pm, then snack two should be close to 3 pm. Snack three should be near 5 pm and dinner would follow near 7 pm.
2. You should not skip breakfast regardless of when you begin your day. Skipping breakfast will result in higher fasting blood glucose and the likelihood of overeating later in the day. Do not use snack one in place of breakfast.
3. You should not skip snacks. If you are not hungry at a recommended snack time, eat half of the snack. Calories help support energy, provide adequate and continuous nutrients, and help prevent overeating at meals.
4. All meal and snack strategies are interchangeable. If one of the meal or snack choices provided is not to your liking, you may choose another suggestion from any one of the meal or snack strategies for that day.
5. It is important that you do not eat the same thing each day. These meal and snack strategies are intended to provide you with a variety of foods and therefore a variety of necessary vitamins, minerals, fiber, and plant nutrients that collectively help reverse weight related insulin resistant states.
6. Water is encouraged. Since everyone is different, water needs are different. Exercise, temperature, humidity, and food choices make a difference in the amount of water used and therefore needed. General recommendations are to consume between 3 and 4 liters of water per day. Drinking water while snacking is an excellent way to achieve water recommendations.
7. If you consume diet drinks, coffee, or any type of drink made with a sugar substitute, you need to be very careful. They are mild diuretics, which may increase water loss, lead to slight dehydration, and stimulate over eating as a result of their sweet taste.
8. Snacks are controlled for sodium. Low sodium snack foods are used to help prevent further hikes in blood pressure.

Level 3

Day 1

Breakfast	½ cup cooked oatmeal, plain + 4 walnut halves, crushed or whole + **P**
Snack 1	5-6 apple slices, with skin + 2 tablespoons sliced or slivered almonds, unsalted
Lunch	3 ounces tuna, canned in water + 2-3 cups of mixed dark greens (spinach leaves, romaine, arugula, lambs lettuce, or any other type of dark green) + **F**
Snack 2	2 cups lite microwave popcorn or 2 cups air popped popcorn + 2 tablespoons almonds, unsalted Or- 6" whole-wheat tortilla + 1 tablespoon reduced fat peanut butter
Dinner	1/3 cup cooked brown rice + 1 cup steamed spinach + **F + P**
Snack 3	Medium celery stalk (6-7"), cut into pieces + 1 tablespoon peanut butter

	Calories	Carbs (g)	Total Fat (g)	Sat. Fat (g)	Sodium (mg)	Fiber (g)
Breakfast	125	14.5	6	<1	2	2.3
Snack 1	84	9.5	5	<1	1	1.4
Lunch	128	5	1.2	<1	330	2.8
Snack 2	167	15	10	<1	1.2	4.3
Or-						
Snack 2	154	25	6	1	260	3
Dinner	107	20	1	0	127	7
Snack 3	91	7.4	5.3	1	151	2

Day 2

Breakfast	½ cup blueberries, fresh or frozen + ½ whole-wheat English muffin, toasted + **F**
Snack 1	1/3 cup of any whole grain cereal, with 5 or more grams of fiber per serving + 2 tablespoons sliced or slivered almonds, unsalted
Lunch	½ whole-wheat pita stuffed with sliced tomatoes, sliced pepper, sprouts, mushrooms + 3 oz tuna, canned in water + **F**
Snack 2	5-6 apple slices + 1/3 cup non-fat or low-fat cottage cheese Or- 6" whole-wheat tortilla + 1 tablespoon peanut butter
Dinner	1/3 cup cooked brown rice + 2 cups broccoli, steamed + **P** + **F**
Snack 3	6 almonds, dry roasted, unsalted

	Calories	Carbs (g)	Total Fat (g)	Sat. Fat (g)	Sodium (mg)	Fiber (g)
Breakfast	117	23.5	1	<1	215	4.2
Snack 1	121	16	6.5	<1	38	7.2
Lunch	193	20	1.75	<1	459	2.8
Snack 2	79	10	1	<1	228	1
Or-						
Snack 2	154	25	5.75	1	260	2.8
Dinner	153	30	1.5	0	82	10
Snack 3	122	3	9	<1	.5	2

Day 3

Breakfast	½ cup cooked oatmeal + **F**
Snack 1	1 cup diced cantaloupe + 4 walnut halves
Lunch	1/3 cup kidney beans, canned, drained mixed with 2-3 cups of mixed dark greens (spinach leaves, romaine, arugula, lambs lettuce, or any other type of dark green) + **P** + **F**
Snack 2	½ cup soybeans (edamame), boiled, unsalted Or- 1 medium orange + 2 tablespoons sliced or slivered almonds, unsalted
Dinner	1 cup steamed green beans + ½ cup steamed mushrooms + **P** + **F**
Snack 3	2 cups air popped popcorn + 1 tablespoon grated parmesan cheese

	Calories	Carbs (g)	Total Fat (g)	Sat. Fat (g)	Sodium (mg)	Fiber (g)
Breakfast	73	13	1.2	0	1.1	2
Snack 1	110	14.5	5.5	<1	15	1.5
Lunch	94	17	<1	0	250	7.6
Snack 2	127	10	6	<1	13	4
Or-						
Snack 2	132	18	6	<1	0	4
Dinner	49	17	0	0	2	5
Snack 3	79	1	5	3	117	0

Day 4

Breakfast	Whole-wheat tortilla, 6" diameter + 1 tablespoon peanut butter + **P**
Snack 1	3 oz low-fat or non-fat yogurt, plain or fruit flavored + 2 tablespoons crushed walnuts
Lunch	1/3 cup kidney or garbanzo beans mixed with 2-3 cups of dark greens (spinach, romaine, arugula, or any other type of dark green) + **P** + **F**
Snack 2	4 small whole-wheat crackers + 1 tablespoon reduced fat peanut butter Or- 5-6 baby carrots + 1 tablespoon peanut butter
Dinner	½ cup peas, boiled + ½ cup canned or frozen corn, mixed, add butter spray and black pepper + **P** + **F**
Snack 3	1/3 cup low-fat or non-fat cottage cheese + ½ cup sliced strawberries, fresh or frozen

	Calories	Carbs (g)	Total Fat (g)	Sat. Fat (g)	Sodium (mg)	Fiber (g)
Breakfast	154	25	5.75	1	260	2.8
Snack 1	95	8.5	5	<1	51	.8
Lunch	94	17	<1	0	250	7.6
Snack 2	152	15	8	1.5	193	2.5
Or-						
Snack 2	110	9	5.8	1	106	1.9
Dinner	80	17	<1	0	106	3.6
Snack 3	73	8	1.2	<1	229	2

Day 5

Breakfast	½ whole-wheat or rye English muffin + ½ tablespoon peanut butter + **P**
Snack 1	1/3 cup whole grain cereal with 5 or more grams fiber per serving, dry + 2 tablespoons sliced almonds, unsalted
Lunch	Whole-wheat tortilla, 6" diameter + 1/3 cup black beans, roll into tortilla + **F**
Snack 2	1 cup honeydew + 1/3 cup low-fat or non-fat cottage cheese Or- ½ cup soybeans (edamame), boiled, no salt
Dinner	½ whole-wheat pita bread (1 small), stuffed with sprouts, diced tomatoes, cucumber slices, red pepper slices, and mushrooms
Snack 3	2 cups air popped popcorn + 1 tablespoon grated parmesan cheese

	Calories	Carbs (g)	Total Fat (g)	Sat. Fat (g)	Sodium (mg)	Fiber (g)
Breakfast	127	16	3.3	1	255	3
Snack 1	120	16	6.5	<1	38	7.2
Lunch	113	30	1	0	372	6
Snack 2	108	18	6.9	<1	245	1
Or-						
Snack 2	127	10	6	<1	13	4.8
Dinner	193	20	1.75	<1	459	2.8
Snack 3	89	12.25	2.4	1.2	117	2.4

Day 6

Breakfast	4 fluid ounces of low-fat soymilk, plain, vanilla, or chocolate + ½ cup sliced strawberries + **P** + **F**
Snack 1	1/3 cup low-fat or non-fat cottage cheese + ½ cup sliced strawberries, fresh or frozen
Lunch	½ whole-wheat pita bread (1 small) stuffed with sprouts, diced tomatoes, cucumber slices, red pepper slices and mushrooms + **P** + **F**
Snack 2	3 oz tuna, canned in water, drained, roll into lettuce leaf, have 2 Or- 4 whole-wheat crackers + 3 oz tuna, in water, drained
Dinner	1/3 cup cooked barley + 1/3 cup kidney beans, mixed, add black pepper + **P** + **F**
Snack 3	Medium celery stalk (6-7"), cut into pieces + 1 tablespoon reduced fat peanut butter

	Calories	Carbs (g)	Total Fat (g)	Sat. Fat (g)	Sodium (mg)	Fiber (g)
Breakfast	131	22	3.3	<1	91	2
Snack 1	73	8	1.2	<1	229	2
Lunch	193	20	1.75	<1	459	2.8
Snack 2	103	1	<1	0	289	.3
Or-						
Snack 2	170	11	1.1	<1	392	1.6
Dinner	144	25	<1	0	170	6.6
Snack 3	90	8	5.7	1	140	2

Day 7

Breakfast	3 ounces non-fat yogurt + ½ cup blueberries, fresh or frozen + **F**
Snack 1	½ cup blueberries, fresh or frozen + 1/3 cup non-fat or low-fat cottage cheese
Lunch	Whole-wheat tortilla, 6' diameter + 2 tablespoons hummus + **P**
Snack 2	Medium orange + 4 walnut halves Or- 5-6 baby carrots + 1 tablespoon reduced fat peanut butter
Dinner	1/3 cup cooked brown rice + 1 cup spinach, boiled/steamed + **P** + **F**
Snack 3	6 almonds or 4 walnut halves, dry roasted, unsalted

	Calories	Carbs (g)	Total Fat (g)	Sat. Fat (g)	Sodium (mg)	Fiber (g)
Breakfast	84	16	<1	0	51	2.4
Snack 1	88	12	1.2	.66	233	2
Lunch	125	23	3.4	<1	290	4.7
Snack 2	113	16.5	5	.45	1	3.3
Or-						
Snack 2	110	9	5.8	1	106	1.9
Dinner	107	20	1	0	127	7
Snack 3	106	3.3	9	1	.5	2

Day 8

Breakfast	½ whole-wheat English muffin, toasted + 1 small orange + **P** + **F**
Snack 1	1 cup honeydew or cantaloupe, diced + 4 walnut halves
Lunch	½ whole-wheat pita bread + 2 tablespoons hummus, add sprouts, diced tomatoes, cucumber slices, red pepper slices and mushrooms + **P** + **F**
Snack 2	½ cup whole grain cereal with 5 or more grams fiber per serving, dry + 2 tablespoons sliced almonds, unsalted Or- ½ cup soybeans (edamame), boiled, no salt
Dinner	1/3 cup cooked brown rice + 2 cups broccoli, steamed, add black pepper + **P** + **F**
Snack 3	3-4 apple slices + low sodium cheese (1 oz)

	Calories	Carbs (g)	Total Fat (g)	Sat. Fat (g)	Sodium (mg)	Fiber (g)
Breakfast	128	29	<1	0	210	5.2
Snack 1	111	16.5	5.25	<1	18	1.3
Lunch	149	24	3.5	<1	292	6
Snack 2	120	16	6.5	<1	38	7.2
Or-						
Snack 2	127	10	6	<1	13	4.8
Dinner	153	30	1.5	0	82	10
Snack 3	110	9	5.25	3	5	1

Day 9

Breakfast	½ cup blueberries, fresh or frozen + 3 ounces non-fat yogurt + **P** + **F**
Snack 1	1/3 cup non-fat or low-fat yogurt, plain or fruit flavored + 2 tablespoons sliced/slivered almonds
Lunch	5-6 baby carrots + 2 tablespoons hummus + **P** + **F**
Snack 2	½ cup sliced strawberries, fresh + 6 almonds, dry roasted, unsalted Or- 3 cups air popped popcorn or 2 cups lite microwave popcorn + 4 walnut halves
Dinner	½ cup mashed sweet potato, add black pepper, cinnamon and butter spray + **P** + **F**
Snack 3	½ cup sliced strawberries, fresh + 1/3 cup non-fat or low-fat cottage cheese

	Calories	Carbs (g)	Total Fat (g)	Sat. Fat (g)	Sodium (mg)	Fiber (g)
Breakfast	84	16	<1	0	51	2.4
Snack 1	114	9	6	<1	50	1.75
Lunch	81	8	4.75	<1	137	2.9
Snack 2	106	10	10	<1	1.3	4
Or-						
Snack 2	113	13.5	5.6	<1	1.4	2.6
Dinner	89	21	<1	0	12	1.5
Snack 3	73	8	1.2	<1	229	2

Day 10

Breakfast	½ cup cooked oatmeal + 4 fluid ounces of low-fat soymilk, plain, vanilla or chocolate + **P** + **F**
Snack 1	1/3 cup whole grain cereal, with 5 or more grams fiber per serving, dry + 2 tablespoons sliced/slivered almonds, unsalted
Lunch	½ whole-wheat pita + 3 oz tuna, canned in water, lettuce, tomato, and cucumber slices + **F**
Snack 2	½ cup soybeans (edamame), boiled, no salt Or- 5-6 apple slices + low sodium cheese (1 oz)
Dinner	1/3 cup cooked brown rice + 1 cup spinach, steamed, add butter spray + **P** + **F**
Snack 3	2 cups air popped popcorn + 1 tablespoon grated parmesan cheese

	Calories	Carbs (g)	Total Fat (g)	Sat. Fat (g)	Sodium (mg)	Fiber (g)
Breakfast	120	16	6.5	<1	38	7.2
Snack 1	120	16	6.5	.5	38	7.2
Lunch	191	20	1.7	<1	457	2.3
Snack 2	127	10	6	<1	13	4.8
Or-						
Snack 2	110	9	5.25	3	5	1
Dinner	107	20	1	0	127	7
Snack 3	90	12.25	2.6	1.2	117	2.4

Day 11

Breakfast	Whole-wheat tortilla, (6" diameter) + 1 tablespoon peanut butter + **P**
Snack 1	½ cup sliced strawberries, fresh + 1/3 cup non-fat or low-fat cottage cheese
Lunch	1/3 cup kidney or garbanzo beans mixed with 2-3 cups of dark greens (spinach leaves, romaine, arugula, lambs lettuce, or any other type of dark green) + **P** + **F**
Snack 2	1 cup honeydew or cantaloupe, diced + 6 almonds, unsalted Or- Medium celery stalk (6-7"), cut into pieces + 1 tablespoon peanut butter
Dinner	½ cup peas, boiled + 1/3 cup brown rice, add black pepper + **P** + **F**
Snack 3	5-6 red pepper slices + 5-6 cucumber slices + 2 tablespoons lite Italian dressing

	Calories	Carbs (g)	Total Fat (g)	Sat. Fat (g)	Sodium (mg)	Fiber (g)
Breakfast	154	25	6	1	260	3
Snack 1	73	8	1.2	<1	229	2
Lunch	94	17	<1	0	250	7.6
Snack 2	132	18	6	<1	0	4
Or-						
Snack 2	90	8	5.7	1	140	2
Dinner	106	22	<1	0	2	3.6
Snack 3	37	3	3	<1	87	.4

Day 12

Breakfast	½ cup blueberries, fresh or frozen + 3 ounces non-fat yogurt + **P** + **F**
Snack 1	¼ cup low-fat cottage cheese + 1 cup honeydew or cantaloupe
Lunch	5-6 baby carrots + 2 tablespoons hummus + **P** + **F**
Snack 2	½ cup blueberries, fresh or frozen + 4 walnut halves Or- 3 oz tuna, canned in water, drained, roll into lettuce leaf, add 1 teaspoon mustard
Dinner	1/3 cup cooked brown rice + 1 cup spinach, steamed + **P** + **F**
Snack 3	3 oz tuna, canned in water, drained, roll into lettuce leaf, add 1 teaspoon mustard

	Calories	Carbs (g)	Total Fat (g)	Sat. Fat (g)	Sodium (mg)	Fiber (g)
Breakfast	84	16	<1	0	51	2.4
Snack 1	88	12	1.2	<1	233	2
Lunch	81	8	4.75	<1	137	2.9
Snack 2	92	11.5	5.5	<1	1.6	2.3
Or-						
Snack 2	103	1	<1	<1	352	.3
Dinner	107	20	1	0	127	7
Snack 3	103	1	<1	<1	352	.3

Day 13

Breakfast	½ cup cooked oatmeal + 4 fluid ounces of low-fat soymilk, plain, vanilla or chocolate + **P** + **F**
Snack 1	Whole-wheat tortilla (6") + 1 tablespoon peanut butter
Lunch	1/3 cup kidney or garbanzo beans mixed with 2-3 cups of dark greens (spinach leaves, romaine, arugula, or any other type of dark green) + **P** + **F**
Snack 2	5-6 baby carrots mixed with 5-6 red pepper slices + 2 tablespoons lite Italian dressing Or- ½ cup soybeans (edamame), boiled, no salt
Dinner	½ cup peas, boiled + 2 cups broccoli, steamed, add black pepper, butter spray + **P** + **F**
Snack 3	6 almonds or 4 walnut halves, dry roasted, unsalted

	Calories	Carbs (g)	Total Fat (g)	Sat. Fat (g)	Sodium (mg)	Fiber (g)
Breakfast	180	29	4	1	91	2
Snack 1	154	25	5.75	1	260	2.8
Lunch	94	17	<1	0	250	7.6
Snack 2	52	6	3.2	<1	254	1
Or-						
Snack 2	127	10	6	<1	13	4.8
Dinner	117	24	<1	0	82	11.6
Snack 3	52	1.5	5	<1	1	.3

Day 14

Breakfast	6" whole-wheat tortilla + 1 tablespoon peanut butter + **P**
Snack 1	5-6 apple slices + 1 tablespoon reduced fat peanut butter
Lunch	½ whole-wheat pita bread + 2 tablespoons hummus, add sprouts, diced tomatoes, cucumber slices, red pepper slices and mushrooms + **P** + **F**
Snack 2	½ cup sliced strawberries, fresh or frozen + 1/3 cup non-fat or low-fat cottage cheese Or- 5-6 baby carrots mixed with 5-6 red pepper slices + 2 tablespoons lite Italian dressing
Dinner	½ cup mashed sweet potato, add black pepper, cinnamon and butter spray + **P** + **F**
Snack 3	1/3 cup sliced strawberries, fresh or frozen + 1/3 cup non-fat or low-fat cottage cheese

	Calories	Carbs (g)	Total Fat (g)	Sat. Fat (g)	Sodium (mg)	Fiber (g)
Breakfast	154	25	5.75	1	260	2.8
Snack 1	102	10	6	<1	0	2
Lunch	149	24	3.5	<1	292	6
Snack 2	73	8	1.2	<1	229	2
Or-						
Snack 2	52	6	3.2	<1	254	1
Dinner	89	21	<1	0	12	1.5
Snack 3	132	17	5.2	<1	0	4.2

Level 4 Weight Related Insulin Resistant Food Strategy

Levels four, five, and six do more than help you lose weight and optimize cardiovascular health. They are optimal food strategies for reversing and managing insulin resistance and related conditions. Don't forget to read the highlights of each level. Here are the general ideas used in planning your next three food strategies. They include the following.

- Whole grains in place of refined carbohydrate sources
- Wide variety of vegetables
- Antioxidant rich fruit
- Two to three servings of dairy
- No more than 6 ounces of animal protein such as meat, poultry, or fish/day*
- Nuts, seeds, and legumes
- Limited total fat coming from spreads and oils

   slightly more animal protein (1-2 ounces/day) is used when calorie levels reach 1,700 and 1,800 calories

Here are the specifics used in planning your next three strategies.

Specific Fat Profile

Total fat intake will be 25%-35% of total calories. Here's your fat percent break down.
- Up to 20% of total fat calories from monounsaturated fats (mufas)
- Up to 10% of total fat calories from polyunsaturated fats (pufas)
- Less than 5% of total fat calories from saturated fat (sat fat)
- Less than 1% of total fat calories from trans-fats
- Dietary cholesterol averages less than 100 milligrams per day, in all three levels!

Here's a Reminder Why Your Fat Profile Needs to be Very Specific
- Mufa's will not lower your HDL or "good" cholesterol
- Mufa's and pufa's help lower your total and LDL cholesterol
- Fatty fish such as salmon, trout, pollock, and halibut contain omega 3 pufas, which have excellent blood triglyceride lowering benefits
- Sat fat worsens insulin resistance and raises you LDL or "bad" cholesterol

- Nuts and seeds are very low in sat fat, good sources of pufas, and cholesterol free

Specific Carbohydrate (carb) Profile

<u>Total carb intake will be 45%-55% of total calories. Here's your carb breakdown.</u>
- All grain products such as oatmeal, rice, pasta, and bread will be whole grains
- Vegetables will provide adequate vitamins and minerals, fiber, and water
- Vegetables are the best sources of phytonutrients, compounds that help fight disease
- All fruit is controlled for quantity and quality
- Dairy such as milk and yogurt will be either fat free or low-fat to minimize total and saturated fat calories along with dietary cholesterol

Here's a Reminder Why Your Carb Profile Needs to be Very Specific
- Carbohydrates are your primary source of fuel
- You need approximately half of your daily calories in the form of carbs
- Benefits of whole grain carbs;
    Vitamins and minerals
    Fiber
    Antioxidants
    Low in added sugars
    Very low is saturated fat
    Contain zero cholesterol
    Help prevent high blood glucose and blood pressure
- The majority of the vegetables you will eat are non-starchy and full of vitamins, minerals, fiber, water, and low in calories. Non-fat and low-fat milk and yogurt are essential foods for weight management, glucose, and blood pressure management

Specific Protein Profile

Total protein intake will be 15%-20% of total calories. Here's your protein breakdown.
- All animal sources will be lean (2-3 grams fat/serving) or very lean (1 gram fat/serving)
- Fresh fish will make up at least two meals per week
- Soy protein and soy products (plant protein) will be used in place of animal protein to help minimize total fat, saturated fat, and dietary cholesterol

Here's a Reminder Why Your Protein Profile Needs to be Very Specific
- Lean and very lean proteins are lowest in calories and total and saturated fat, which help lower total and LDL cholesterol
- Fish is not only an excellent source of protein; certain types of fish contain omega 3 fats, which have excellent heart and artery protective features
- Consuming soy protein will improve your blood cholesterol and provide adequate dietary fiber, an essential component in managing blood glucose

LEVEL FOUR HIGHLIGHTS

Cal Avg	Carb	Fiber	Protein	Total fat	Mufa	Pufa	Sat fat	Trans fat	Diet. Cholesterol
1241	49%	28	19%	30%	16%	8%	5%	0%	48

Fiber, protein, monounsaturated fat (mufa), polyunsaturated fat (pufa), sat fat, trans-fat measured in grams (g). Dietary cholesterol measured in milligrams (mg)

Jerrod P. Libonati, MS, RD

Level 4

Day 1

Breakfast	Whole wheat toast	1 slice
	Benecol Light	2 tsp
	Strawberries, sliced, fresh/frozen	½ cup
	Non-fat yogurt, plain/flavored	6 oz
	Coffee	12 fl oz, 2 tsp nf milk
Snack	Low-fat/low-sodium cottage cheese	1/3 cup
	Water	12 fl oz
	Coffee	8 fl oz, 2 tsp nf milk
Lunch	Rye bread	1 slice
	Tuna in water, low-sodium, Albacore	3 oz
	Tomato slices	3 slices
	Chopped celery and avocado	2 Tbsp each
	Orange	1 medium

Mix avocado, chopped celery, open face sandwich, add tomato

Snack	Non-fat yogurt, plain/flavored	6 oz
	Banana	4" small
	Sesame seeds, unsalted	2 Tbsp
	Water	16 fl oz
Dinner	Brown rice	1/3 cup cooked
	Halibut, baked, grilled, broiled, add herbs	3 oz
	Large Salad	
	Spinach, fresh, raw + mixed greens	2 cups each
	Tomato/cucumber slices	6 slices total
	Salad dressing, lite + olive oil	2 Tbsp, 1 Tbsp
	Broccoli, steamed, no salt	1.5 cups

Add fresh lemon to fish, drizzle olive oil on broccoli, add black pepper, salt free seasonings

Add Calories	1400 Calories	1500 Calories	1600 Calories	1700 Calories	1800 Calories
Breakfast	2 tsp Benecol	2 tsp Benecol .5 c straw	2 tsp Benecol 1 c straw.	2 tsp Benecol 1.5 c straw.	2 tsp Benecol 1.5 c straw.
Snack					
Lunch	1 tsp avocado	2 tsp avocado	2 tsp avocado	2 tsp avocado	2 tsp avocado
Snack	1 tsp seeds		1 tsp seeds	2 tsp seeds	3 tsp seeds
Dinner	1 oz fish 1 tsp oil	2 oz fish 1 tsp oil	3 oz fish 1 tsp oil	3 oz fish 1 tsp oil .5 c broc	4 oz fish 1 tsp oil 1 c broc
Snack					

Day 2

Breakfast	Whole wheat tortilla (6")	1 small
	Peanut butter	1 Tbsp
	Non-fat milk	4 fl. oz
	Strawberries, sliced, fresh/frozen	1 cup
	Coffee	12 fl oz, 2 tsp nf milk
Snack	Non-fat yogurt, plain/flavored	6 oz
	Apple	5-6 slices
	Sesame seeds, unsalted	2 Tbsp
Coffee	8 fl oz, 2 tsp nf milk	
Lunch	Tofu, grilled, stir fry	4 oz
	Brown rice	1/3 cup cooked
	Add salt free seasoning, black pepper	
	Orange	1 medium
	Flaxseeds	1 Tbsp

Use Pam or Wesson Spray to fry tofu, add flax to brown rice

Snack	Soybeans, steamed, unsalted	1 cup
	Water	12 fl oz
Dinner	Chicken breast, no skin, white meat	4 oz (broiled)
	Broccoli, steamed, no salt	1.5 cups
	Extra virgin olive oil	4 tsp
	Add herbs, salt free seasoning, fresh lemon to chicken breast	
	Sweet potato, w/skin (tennis ball in size)	1 each

Drizzle olive oil on broccoli and sweet potato, add cinnamon to sweet potato, salt free seasoning

Snack	Cantaloupe, diced	1 cup

Add Calories	1400 Calories	1500 Calories	1600 Calories	1700 Calories	1800 Calories
Breakfast	.5 c straw	.5 c straw	1 c straw	1.5 c straw	1.5 c straw
Snack			1 tsp seeds	2 tsp seeds	2 tsp seeds
Lunch			1/3 c rice	1/3 c rice	2/3 c rice
Snack					
Dinner	.5 c broccoli	1 c broccoli 1 tsp oil	1 c broccoli 1 tsp oil	1 oz chick. 1.5 c broccoli 1 tsp oil	2 oz chick. 1.5 c broccoli 1 tsp oil
Snack		.5 c cant.	.5 c cant.	.5 c cant.	.5 c cant.

Day 3

Breakfast	Oatmeal, steel cut/whole oats	½ cup
	Sliced almonds, unsalted	1 Tbsp
	Benecol Light	1 Tbsp
	Blueberries, fresh/frozen	½ cup
	Non fat milk	4 fl. oz
	Coffee	12 fl oz, 2 tsp nf milk
Snack	Non-fat yogurt, plain/flavored	6 oz
	Orange	5-6 pieces
Coffee	8 fl oz, 2 tsp nf milk	
Lunch	Kidney beans	1/3 cup
	Brown rice	¾ cup cooked
	Add salt free seasoning, black pepper, cilantro	
	Extra virgin olive oil	2 tsp
	Water	16 fl oz
Snack	Kiwi	4 slices
	Walnut halves, unsalted	2 tsp crushed
	Water	16 fl oz
Dinner	Salmon, fresh/farmed (baked/broiled/grilled)	3 oz
	Summer squash, baked, no salt	2 cups
	Olive oil, drizzle over squash	2 tsp
	Add ground cinnamon, black pepper, salt free seasonings	
Snack	Non-fat yogurt, plain/flavored	6 oz

Add Calories	1400 Calories	1500 Calories	1600 Calories	1700 Calories	1800 Calories
Breakfast		½ c berries	½ c berries 2 tsp almonds	½ c berries 2 tsp almonds	1 c berries 2 tsp almonds
Snack			4 pieces orange	4 pieces orange	4 pieces orange
Lunch		1 tsp oil	1 tsp oil	1 tsp oil	1 tsp oil
Snack		2 slices kiwi	2 slices kiwi	2 slices kiwi	2 slices kiwi
Dinner	2 tsp oil	2 tsp oil	1 oz fish 2 tsp oil	2 oz fish 2 tsp oil	3 oz fish 2 tsp oil
Snack				2 tsp almonds	2 tsp almonds

Day 4

Breakfast	Whole grain cereal	½ cup
	Non-fat milk	4 fl. oz
	Flax seeds	1 Tbsp
	Sliced almonds, unsalted	1 Tbsp
	Coffee	12 fl oz, 2 tsp nf milk
Snack	Baby carrots	10 each
	Hummus, plain/flavored	2 Tbsp
	Coffee	8 fl oz, 2 tsp nf milk
	Water	12 fl oz
Lunch	Loose leaf lettuce	3 leafs (med-large)
	Tuna in water, low-sodium, Albacore	3 oz
	Tomato slices/chopped celery	3 slices/2 tbsp
	Canola oil	2 tsp
	Kiwi	8 slices

Mix tuna in oil, add chopped celery, open face sandwich, add tomato slices

Snack	Popcorn, microwave lite, less salt	3 cups popped
	Water	16 fl oz
Dinner	Tofu, grilled/stir fry	4 oz
	Spinach, steamed, no salt	1 cup cooked
	Brown rice	½ cup cooked

Add curry seasoning to tofu with basil, stir fry tofu in Pam or Wesson Spray, salt free seasoning

Snack	Watermelon, diced/cubed	2 cups

Add Calories	1400 Calories	1500 Calories	1600 Calories	1700 Calories	1800 Calories
Breakfast		1 tsp almonds	½ c cereal 2 tsp almonds	½ c cereal 2 tsp almonds	½ c cereal 2 oz milk 2 tsp almonds
Snack		1 Tbsp hummus	1 Tbsp hummus	1 Tbsp hummus	1 Tbsp hummus
Lunch					1 tsp oil
Snack		4 slices kiwi	4 slices kiwi	4 slices kiwi	4 slices kiwi
Dinner	1/2 c rice	1 oz tofu ½ cup rice	1 oz tofu ½ cup rice	1 oz tofu 1 cup rice	2 oz tofu 1 cup rice
Snack					

Jerrod P. Libonati, MS, RD

Day 5

Breakfast	Rye bread toasted	1 slice
	Benecol Light	2 tsp
	Cottage cheese, low-sodium, low-fat	1/3 cup
	Coffee	12 fl oz, 2 tsp nf milk
Snack	Whole wheat English muffin	½ each
	Peanut butter	1 Tbsp
	Coffee	8 fl oz, 2 tsp nf milk
Lunch	Large Salad	

Spinach leaves, fresh, raw		2 cups
	Salad greens	2 cups
	Tomato slices/chopped celery	3 slices/2 Tbsp
	Garbanzo beans, drained, rinsed	1/3 cup
	Salad dressing, lite	2 tbsp

Mix beans, chopped celery and tomato slices

Snack	Non-fat yogurt, plain/flavored	6 oz
	Banana	4" small
	Water	16 fl oz
Dinner	Chicken breast, white meat/no skin	3 oz (baked, broiled)
	Cooked lentils & barley	1/4 cup and 1/3 cup
	Extra virgin olive oil	1 Tbsp

Add fresh lemon to chicken, drizzle olive oil on lentil/barley mix, add black pepper, salt free seasoning

Snack	Kiwi	4 slices
	Almonds, sliced, unsalted	2 Tbsp
	Water	16 fl oz

Add Calories	1400 Calories	1500 Calories	1600 Calories	1700 Calories	1800 Calories
Breakfast			1 tsp Benecol	1 tsp Benecol	1 tsp Benecol
Snack					1 tsp p butter
Lunch			1/3 c beans	1/3 c beans	2/3 c beans
Snack					
Dinner	1 tsp oil	2 tsp oil ¼ c lentils	2 tsp oil ¼ c lentils	3 tsp oil ¼ c lentils 1/3 c barley	3 tsp oil ¼ c lentils 1/3 c barley
Snack	4 slices kiwi	4 slices kiwi	4 slices kiwi 2 tsp almonds	4 slices kiwi 2 tsp almonds	4 slices kiwi 2 tsp almonds

Day 6

Breakfast	Non-fat yogurt, plain/flavored	6 oz
	Flaxseeds	1 Tbsp
	Blueberries, fresh/frozen	½ cup
	Coffee	12 fl oz, 2 tsp nf milk
Snack	Oatmeal, instant pkg, plain	½ packet
	Almonds, sliced, unsalted	2 Tbsp
	Apple slices	5-6 slices
	Coffee	8 fl oz, 2 tsp nf milk
Lunch	Tofu, grilled or baked	3 oz
	Brown rice	1/3 cup cooked
	Strawberries, sliced, fresh/frozen	1 cup

Add basil and curry to tofu; use Pam or Wesson spray to grill or stir fry tofu

Snack	Non-fat yogurt, plain/flavored	6 oz
	Kiwi, fresh	4 slices
	Water	16 fl oz
Dinner	Salmon, fresh/farmed (baked, broiled, grilled)	3 oz
	Broccoli, steamed, no salt	2 cups
	Sweet potato w/skin	1 (tennis ball size)
	Extra virgin olive oil	1 Tbsp

Add fresh lemon to fish, drizzle olive oil on broccoli, add cinnamon, black pepper, salt free seasoning

Snack	Sesame seeds, unsalted	2 Tbsp
	Water	16 fl oz

Add Calories	1400 Calories	1500 Calories	1600 Calories	1700 Calories	1800 Calories
Breakfast				½ c berries	½ c berries
Snack				2 tsp almonds	2 tsp almonds
Lunch		2 oz tofu	2 oz tofu 1/3 c rice	3 oz tofu 1/3 c rice	3 oz tofu 1/3 c rice
Snack	4 slices kiwi	4 slices kiwi	4 slices kiwi	4 slices kiwi	4 slices kiwi
Dinner		1 tsp oil	1 tsp oil	1 tsp oil	2 oz salmon 1 tsp oil
Snack			2 tsp seeds	2 tsp seeds	

Jerrod P. Libonati, MS, RD

Day 7

Breakfast	Rye bread, toasted/ peanut butter	1 slice/2 tsp
	Non-fat milk	4 fl oz
	Coffee	12 fl oz, 2 tsp nf milk
Snack	Non-fat yogurt/flaxseeds	6 oz container/1 tbsp
	Water	12 fl oz
	Coffee	8 fl oz, 2 tsp nf milk
Lunch	Whole wheat tortilla	1 small (6")
	Tuna in water, low-sodium, Albacore	3 oz
	Lettuce leaf/avocado	2 loose/2 Tbsp
	Tomato slices/chopped celery	3 slices/2 Tbsp
	Orange	1 medium

Mix avocado, chopped celery, tomato slices to make open face sandwich

Snack	Banana/Walnut halves	4" small/6 halves
	Water	16 fl oz
Dinner	Tofu, grilled/stir fry	3 oz
	Spinach, stir fry	1 cup
	Olive oil	1 Tbsp
	Brown rice, kidney beans	1/3 cup cooked

Stir fry tofu with Pam or Wesson spray, add olive oil to spinach and rice and beans
Add black pepper, salt free seasonings to brown rice and beans

Snack	Non-fat yogurt, plain/flavored	6 oz

Add Calories	1400 Calories	1500 Calories	1600 Calories	1700 Calories	1800 Calories
Breakfast					
Snack		2 tsp p butter 2 tsp flaxseeds	2 tsp p butter 2 tsp flaxseeds	2 tsp p butter 2 tsp flaxseeds	2 tsp p butter 2 tsp flaxseeds
Lunch			3 tsp avocado	3 tsp avocado 1 oz tuna	3 tsp avocado 1 oz tuna
Snack		4 w halves	4 w halves	4 w halves	4 w halves
Dinner	1 oz tofu 1/3 c beans	1 oz tofu 1/3 c beans	1 oz tofu 1/3 c rice 1/3 c beans	3 oz tofu 1/3 c rice 1/3 c beans	3 oz tofu ½ c spinach 2/3 c rice 1/3 c beans
Snack					

Level 5 Weight Related Insulin Resistant Food Strategy

Level five is your first food strategy designed at educating you on controlling unhealthy blood glucose. To accomplish this, you will begin learning how to;
- Identify carbs
- Control carbs
- Space carbs
- Begin using the Diabetic Exchange

The diabetic exchange system is a simple way for you to identify and control the total amount of carbohydrate (total grams) you consume at snacks and meals. The name is misleading as it's not a system only for diabetics. Rather, it's a guide to help <u>everyone</u> control and manage their carb intake. In essence, it teaches you how to eat and drink approximately the same amount of carb at snacks and meals. By learning this counting method, you prevent more than calorie overload, you prevent blood glucose surges! Your pancreas doesn't have to work overtime producing and shipping unnecessary concentrations of insulin into the blood. By controlling the portion of carb you consume, your arteries are not subjected to the hyperglycemic and hyperinsulinemic states.

The diabetic exchange is therefore a great tool for everyone to use as it creates a limit at snacks, meals, and total carbs consumed throughout the day each and everyday. It's a quick and easy way for you to manage carb grams and calories from carbs. All of this is detailed for you step by step over seven days worth of examples.

Day one is your guide. It's broken down over four pages allowing you to see how the food strategies are implemented. All remaining days follow the same pattern, but are condensed into two pages. The food strategy listed provides you with approximately 1,200-1,300 calories. All other calorie levels are listed in the table at the bottom of the page.

LEVEL FIVE HIGHLIGHTS

- Carbs underlined
- Total carbs identified
- Diabetic exchange identified
- Carbs are evenly spaced throughout the day
- Average carbohydrates per meal/snack   26 grams/17 grams
- Average fiber per day   28 grams
- Total Fat % Average per day   30%
     Mufa fat % average   16%
     Pufa fat % average   8%
     Sat fat % average   5%
     Trans-fat % average   <1%
- Average dietary cholesterol intake per day   <50 milligrams!

Level 5 Step I

Day 1

Breakfast	Blueberries, fresh/frozen	½ cup
	Cantaloupe, diced/cubed	1 cup
	Walnut halves	6 halves
	Coffee	12 fl oz, 2 tsp nf milk
Snack	Whole wheat English muffin	½ each
	Reduced fat peanut butter	2 tsp
	Non-fat milk	4 fl oz
	Coffee	8 fl oz, 2 tsp nf milk
Lunch	Chicken breast, white meat, no skin	3 oz (baked, broiled)
	Large Salad	
	Spinach, fresh & salad greens	2 cups each
	Garbanzo beans, drained/rinsed	1/3 cup
	Tomato & cucumber slices	3-4 slices each
	Salad dressing, lite	2 Tbsp
	Water	16 fl oz

Mix greens, beans, tomato, & cucumber w/dressing; add salt free seasoning, black pepper

Snack	Baby carrots	8 each
	Hummus, regular/flavored	2 Tbsp
	Water	16 fl oz
Dinner	Halibut, baked, grilled, broiled	3 oz
	Broccoli, steamed, no salt	1.5 cups
	Benecol light	1 Tbsp
	Sweet potato, w/skin (tennis ball in size)	1 each
	Extra virgin olive oil	1 tbsp

Add fresh lemon, Benecol, olive oil, black pepper, & salt free seasoning

Snack	Apple w/skin	1 small

You Need to Know

Carbohydrates are underlined. Other foods may contain carbohydrates, but are not classified as carbs. Notice each meal or snack provides you with some carbohydrate. Turn the page.

Jerrod P. Libonati, MS, RD

Level 5 Step II

Day 1

Breakfast	<u>Blueberries, fresh/frozen</u>	½ cup (1/2 carb)
	<u>Cantaloupe, diced/cubed</u>	1 cup (1 carb)
	Walnut halves	6 halves
	Coffee	12 fl oz, 2 tsp nf milk

Total Carbs 24 grams or the approximate equivalent to 2 Diabetic exchanges

Snack	<u>Whole wheat English muffin</u>	½ each (1 carb)
	Reduced fat peanut butter	2 tsp
	<u>Non-fat milk</u>	4 fl oz (1/2 carb)
	Coffee	8 fl oz, 2 tsp nf milk

Total Carbs 20 grams or the approximate equivalent to 1.5 Diabetic exchanges

Lunch	Chicken breast, white meat, no skin	3 oz (baked, broiled)
	Large Salad	
	<u>Spinach & salad greens</u>	2 cups each
	<u>Garbanzo beans,</u> drained, rinsed	1/3 cup (1 carb)
	<u>Tomato & cucumber slices</u>	3-4 slices each
	Salad dressing, lite	2 Tbsp
	Water	16 fl oz

Mix greens, beans, tomato & cucumber w/dressing; add salt free seasoning, black pepper
Total Carbs 26 grams or the approximate equivalent of 2 Diabetic exchanges

Snack	<u>Baby carrots</u>	8 each (½ carb)
	<u>Hummus</u>, regular/flavored	2 Tbsp (½ carb)
	Water	16 fl oz

Total Carbs 12 grams or the approximate equivalent of 1 Diabetic exchange

Dinner	Halibut, baked, grilled, broiled	3 oz
	<u>Broccoli, steamed,</u> no salt	1.5 cups (1 carb)
	Benecol light	1 Tbsp
	<u>Sweet potato, w/skin</u> (tennis ball in size)	1 each (1 carb)
	Extra virgin olive oil	1 Tbsp

Add fresh lemon, Benecol, olive oil, black pepper & salt free seasoning
Total Carbs 28 grams or the approximate equivalent of 2 Diabetic exchanges

Snack	<u>Apple w/skin</u>	1 small (1 carb)
	Water	16 fl oz

Total Carbs 16 grams or the approximate equivalent of 1Diabetic exchange

You Need to Know

Carbohydrates are underlined. Total grams of carbs noted under each meal or snack. Total carb grams plus diabetic exchange helps manage your total daily carb intake. Approximately 15 grams of total carbohydrate equals one carbohydrate (1 carb). One carb equals one exchange. Goal is to keep total carb intake (total grams or exchanges) relatively even at meals or snacks. Turn the page.

Level 5 Step III

Day 1

Breakfast	Blueberries, fresh/frozen	½ cup (1/2 carb)
	Cantaloupe, diced/cubed	1 cup (1 carb)
	Walnut halves	6 halves
	Coffee	12 fl oz, 2 tsp nf milk

Total Carbs 24 grams or the approximate equivalent to 2 Diabetic exchanges

Snack	Whole wheat English muffin	½ each (1 carb)
	Reduced fat peanut butter	2 tsp
	Non-fat milk	4 fl oz (1/2 carb)
	Coffee	8 fl oz, 2 tsp nf milk

Total Carbs 20 grams or the approximate equivalent to 1.5 Diabetic exchanges

Lunch	Chicken breast, white meat, no skin	3 oz (baked, broiled)
	Large Salad	
	Spinach, fresh & salad greens	2 cups each
	Garbanzo beans, drained, rinsed	1/3 cup (1 carb)
	Tomato & cucumber slices	3-4 slices each
	Salad dressing, lite	2 Tbsp
	Water	16 fl oz

Mix greens, beans, tomato, & cucumber w/dressing; add salt free seasoning & black pepper
Total Carbs 26 grams or the approximate equivalent of 2 Diabetic exchanges

Snack	Baby carrots	8 each (½ carb)
	Hummus, regular/flavored	2 Tbsp (½ carb)
	Water	16 fl oz

Total Carbs 12 grams or the approximate equivalent of 1 Diabetic exchange

Dinner	Halibut, baked, grilled, broiled	3 oz
	Broccoli, steamed, no salt	1.5 cups (1 carb)
	Benecol light	1 Tbsp
	Sweet potato, w/skin (tennis ball in size)	1 each (1 carb)
	Extra virgin olive oil	1 Tbsp

Add fresh lemon, Benecol, olive oil, black pepper, & salt free seasoning
Total Carbs 28 grams or the approximate equivalent of 2 Diabetic exchanges

Snack	Apple w/skin	1 small (1 carb)
	Water	16 fl oz

Total Carbs 16 grams or the approximate equivalent of 1 Diabetic exchange

Spacing Your Carbs

Breakfast	2	(approximately 30 grams total carb)
Snack	1.5	(more than 15, near 23 grams total carb)
Lunch	2	(approximately 30 grams total carb)
Snack	1	(approximately 15 grams total carb)
Dinner	2	(approximately 30 grams total carb)
Snack	1	(approximately 15 grams total carb)

Notice your total carb intake was relatively stable throughout the day. You did not skip meals or snacks. Snacks have fewer total carbs compared to meals, but enough to prevent large fluctuations in blood glucose. Great job!

Level 5 Step IV

Day 1

Meal	Food	Amount
Breakfast	Blueberries, fresh/frozen	½ cup (1/2 carb)
	Cantaloupe, diced/cubed	1 cup (1 carb)
	Walnut halves, unsalted	6 halves
	Coffee	12 fl oz, 2 tsp nf milk
Snack	Whole wheat English muffin	½ each (1 carb)
	Reduced fat peanut butter	2 tsp
	Non-fat milk	4 fl oz (1 carb)
	Coffee	8 fl oz, 2 tsp nf milk
Lunch	Chicken breast, white meat, no skin	3 oz (baked, broiled)
	Large Salad	
	Spinach, fresh & Salad greens	2 cups each
	Garbanzo beans, drained, rinsed	1/3 cup (1 carb)
	Tomato & cucumber slices	3-4 slices each
	Salad dressing, lite	2 Tbsp
	Water	16 fl oz

Mix greens, beans, tomato, & cucumber into dressing; add salt free seasoning to chick breast

Meal	Food	Amount
Snack	Baby carrots	8 each (1/2 carb)
	Hummus, regular/flavored	2 Tbsp (1/2 carb)
	Water	16 fl oz
Dinner	Halibut, baked, grilled, broiled	3 oz
	Broccoli, steamed, no salt	1.5 cups (1 carb)
	Benecol light	1 Tbsp
	Sweet potato, w/skin (tennis ball in size)	1 small (1 carb)
	Extra virgin olive oil	1 Tbsp

Add fresh lemon, Benecol, olive oil, black pepper & salt free seasoning

Meal	Food	Amount
Snack	Apple w/skin	1 medium (1 carb)
	Water	16 fl oz

Add Calories	1400 Calories	1500 Calories	1600 Calories	1700 Calories	1800 Calories
Breakfast	½ c berries	½ c berries 1 tsp Benecol	½ c berries 1 tsp Benecol	1 c berries 1 tsp Benecol 4 fl oz milk	1 c berries 2 tsp Benecol 4 fl oz milk
Snack					
Lunch	1/3 c beans	1/3 c beans	1/3 c beans	1/3 c beans	1/3 c beans
Snack					
Dinner		1 oz fish 1 tsp oil	2 oz fish 2 tsp oil	2 oz fish 2 tsp oil	3 oz fish 3 tsp oil
Snack					

Day 2

Breakfast
- Oatmeal, steel cut, whole oats — ½ cup (1 carb)
- Benecol light — 2 tsp
- Blueberries, fresh/frozen — ½ cup (1/2 carb)
- Non-fat milk — 4 fl oz (1/2 carb)
- Flaxseeds — 1 Tbsp
- Coffee — 12 fl oz, 2 tsp nf milk

Total Carbs 31 grams or the approximate equivalent of 2 Diabetic exchanges

Snack
- Non-fat yogurt, plain/flavored — 6 oz (1 carb)
- Water — 12 fl oz
- Coffee — 8 fl oz, 2 tsp nf milk

Total Carbs 17 grams or the approximate equivalent of 1 Diabetic exchange

Lunch
- Whole wheat tortilla — 1 small (6") (1 carb)
- Turkey breast, low-sodium — 2 oz
- Avocado — 1 Tbsp
- Tomato slice/Loose leaf lettuce — 3 slices/2 leaves
- Strawberries, sliced, fresh/frozen — 1 cup (1 carb)

Mix avocado, tomato slice, and lettuce into whole wheat tortilla
Total Carbs 26 grams or the approximate equivalent of 2 Diabetic exchanges

Snack
- Soybeans, steamed, no salt — 1 cup (1 carb)
- Apple w/skin — 1 medium (1 carb)
- Water — 16 fl oz

Total Carbs 35 grams or the approximate equivalent of 2 Diabetic exchanges

Dinner
- Chicken breast, white meat, no skin — 2 oz (baked, broiled)
- Broccoli, steamed, no salt — 2 cups (1 carb)
- Brown rice — 1/3 c cooked (1 carb)
- Extra virgin olive oil — 1 Tbsp
- Flaxseeds — 1 Tbsp

Add Benecol to broccoli; olive oil & flaxseeds to brown rice and broccoli
Total Carbs 30 grams or the approximate equivalent of 2 Diabetic exchanges

Snack
- Non-fat milk — 4 fl oz (1/2 carb)
- Almond butter — 2 tsp
- Water — 16 fl oz

Total Carbs 7 grams or the approximate equivalent of ½ Diabetic exchange

You Need to Know

Carbohydrates are underlined. Other foods may contain carbohydrates but are not classified as carbs. Notice each meal or snack provides you with carbohydrate. Total carb grams plus diabetic exchange helps manage your total daily carb intake. Total carbs are distributed evenly throughout the day!

Jerrod P. Libonati, MS, RD

Day 2 Continued

Breakfast	Oatmeal, steel cut, whole oats	½ cup (1 carb)
	Benecol light	2 tsp
	Blueberries, fresh/frozen	½ cup (1/2 carb)
	Non-fat milk	4 fl oz (1/2 carb)
	Flaxseeds	1 Tbsp
	Coffee	12 fl oz, 2 tsp nf milk
Snack	Non-fat yogurt, plain/flavored	6 oz (1 carb)
	Water	12 fl oz
	Coffee	8 fl oz, 2 tsp nf milk
Lunch	Whole wheat tortilla	1 small (6") (1 carb)
	Turkey breast, low-sodium/avocado	2 oz/1 Tbsp
	Tomato slice/Loose leaf lettuce	3 slices/2 leaves
	Loose leaf lettuce	2 leaf
	Strawberries, sliced, fresh/frozen	1 cup (1 carb)

Mix avocado, tomato slice, and lettuce into whole wheat tortilla

Snack	Soybeans, steamed, no salt	1 cup (1 carb)
	Apple w/skin	1 medium (1 carb)
	Water	16 fl oz
Dinner	Chicken breast, white meat, no skin	2 oz (baked, broiled)
	Broccoli, steamed	2 cups (1 carb)
	Brown rice	1/3 c cooked (1 carb)
	Extra virgin olive oil/Flaxseeds	1 Tbsp/1 Tbsp

Add Benecol to broccoli; olive oil & flaxseeds to brown rice and broccoli

Snack	Non-fat milk	4 fl oz (1/2 carb)
	Almond butter/water	2 tsp/16 fl oz

Add Calories	1400 Calories	1500 Calories	1600 Calories	1700 Calories	1800 Calories
Breakfast	1 tsp flax 1 tsp Benecol	1 tsp flax 1 tsp Ben.	1 tsp flax 1 tsp Ben.	1 tsp flax 1 tsp Bene. ½ c berries	1 tsp flax 1 tsp Bene. ½ c berries
Snack					
Lunch	1 Tbsp avo	1 Tbsp avo	1 Tbsp avo	1 Tbsp avo	1 Tbsp avo
Snack					
Dinner		1 oz chicken 1 tsp oil	2 oz chicken 1 tsp oil 1/3 c rice	2 oz chicken 2 tsp oil 1/3 c rice	3 oz chicken 2 tsp oil 1/3 c rice
Snack	1 tsp al. but	2 tsp al. but			2 tsp al. but

Spacing Your Carbs

Breakfast	2	(approximately 30 grams total carb)
Snack	1	(approximately 15 grams total carb)
Lunch	2	(approximately 30 grams total carb)
Snack	2	(approximately 30 grams total carb)
Dinner	2	(approximately 30 grams total carb)
Snack	½	(between 7-9 grams total carb)

What State Do You Live In?

Day 3

Breakfast	<u>Non-fat yogurt, plain/flavored</u>	6 oz (1 carb)
	<u>Blueberries</u>, fresh/frozen	½ cup (1/2 carb)
	<u>Strawberries, sliced</u>,fresh/frozen	½ cup (1/2 carb)
	Chopped walnuts, no salt (add to yogurt)	1 Tbsp
	Coffee	12 fl oz, 2 tsp nf milk

Total Carbs 34 grams or the approximate equivalent of 2 Diabetic exchanges

Snack	<u>Banana</u>	1 small (1 carb)
	Sesame seeds, unsalted	2 tsp
	Water	16 fl oz
	Coffee	8 fl oz, 2 tsp nf milk

Total Carbs 14 grams or the approximate equivalent of 1 Diabetic exchange

Lunch	Large Salad	
	<u>Spinach</u>, raw & <u>Salad</u> greens	2 cups each (1 carb)
	<u>Tomato & cucumber slices</u>	3-4 slices each
	Flaxseeds	1 Tbsp
	<u>Kidney beans</u>, rinsed/drained	1/3 cup (1 carb)
	Extra virgin olive oil	2 tsp
	Salad dressing, lite	2 Tbsp

Mix all ingredients
Total Carbs 27 grams or the approximate equivalent of 2 Diabetic exchanges

Snack	<u>Non-fat yogurt</u>, plain/flavored	6 oz (1 carb)
	Flaxseeds	1 Tbsp
	Water	16 fl oz

Total Carbs 17 grams or the approximate equivalent of 1 Diabetic exchange

Dinner	Salmon, fresh or farmed (baked/grilled/broiled)	2 oz
	<u>Sweet potato w/skin</u> (tennis ball in size)	1 small (1 carb)
	<u>Broccoli</u>, steamed, no salt	1.5 cups (1 carb)
	Extra virgin olive oil	2 tsp
	Benecol light	1 Tbsp

Add fresh lemon, dill, salt free seasoning, benecol, & drizzle olive oil
Total Carbs 37 grams or the approximate equivalent of 2 Diabetic exchanges

Snack	Almond butter	2 tsp
	Water	16 fl oz

You Need to Know

Carbohydrates are underlined. Other foods may contain carbohydrates, but are not classified as carbs. Notice each meal or snack provides you with carbohydrate. Total carb grams plus diabetic exchange helps manage your total daily carb intake. Total carbs are distributed evenly throughout the day!

Day 3 Continued

Breakfast	Non-fat yogurt, plain/flavored	6 oz (1 carb)
	Blueberries, fresh/frozen	½ cup (1/2 carb)
	Strawberries, sliced, fresh/frozen	½ cup (1/2 carb)
	Chopped walnuts, no salt (add to yogurt)	1 Tbsp
	Coffee	12 fl oz, 2 tsp nf milk
Snack	Banana	1 small (1 carb)
	Sesame seeds, unsalted	2 tsp
	Water	12 fl
	Coffee	8 fl oz, 2 tsp nf milk
Lunch	Large Salad	
	Spinach, raw & salad greens	2 cups each (1 carb)
	Tomato & cucumber slices	3-4 slices
	Flaxseeds	1 Tbsp
	Kidney beans, rinsed/drained	1/3 cup (1/3 carb)
	Extra virgin olive oil	2 tsp
	Salad dressing, lite	2 Tbsp

Mix all ingredients

Snack	Non-fat yogurt, plain/flavored	6 oz (1 carb)
	Flaxseeds/water	1 Tbsp/16 fl oz
Dinner	Salmon, fresh/farmed (baked/grilled/broiled)	2 oz
	Sweet potato w/skin (tennis ball in size)	1 small (1 carb)
	Broccoli, steamed, no salt	2 cups (1 carb)
	Extra virgin olive oil/Bencol light	2 tsp/1 Tbsp

Add fresh lemon, dill, salt free seasoning, benecol, & drizzle olive oil

Snack	Almond butter/water	2 tsp/16 fl oz

Add Calories	1400 Calories	1500 Calories	1600 Calories	1700 Calories	1800 Calories
Breakfast		½ c berries 2 tsp nuts	½ c berries 2 tsp nuts	¾ c berries 2 tsp nuts	¾ c berries 2 tsp nuts
Snack					
Lunch	1 tsp oil	2 tsp oil	2 tsp oil	1/3 c beans 2 tsp oil	1/3 c beans 2 tsp oil
Snack					
Dinner	1 oz fish	1 oz fish	2 oz fish 1 tsp oil	2 oz fish 1 tsp oil	3 oz fish 1 tsp oil
Snack					1 tsp al. butter

Spacing Your Carbs

Breakfast	2	(approximately 30 grams total carb)
Snack	1	(approximately 15 grams total carb)
Lunch	2	(approximately 30 grams total carb)
Snack	1	(approximately 15 grams total carb)
Dinner	2	(approximately 30 grams total carb)
Snack	0	(less than 5 grams total carb)

Day 4

Breakfast	<u>Non-fat milk</u>	4 fl oz (½ carb)
	<u>Whole grain cereal</u>	½ cup (1 carb)
	<u>Banana, sliced</u>	small (4") (1 carb)
	Flaxseeds	2 tsp
	Sliced almonds, unsalted	1 tsp
	Coffee	12 fl oz, 2 tsp nf milk

Total Carbs 40 grams or the approximate equivalent of 2.5 Diabetic exchanges

Snack	<u>Whole wheat English muffin</u>	½ each (1 carb)
	Benecol light	2 tsp
	Water	16 fl oz
	Coffee	8 fl oz, 2 tsp nf milk

Total Carbs 13 grams or the approximate equivalent of 1 Diabetic exchange

Lunch	<u>Loose leaf lettuce</u>	2 leaves
	Tuna in water, low-sodium, Albacore	2 oz
	<u>Tomato slices</u>	3-4 slices
	Avocado	2 Tbsp
	<u>Soybeans, steamed, no salt</u>	½ cup (1 carb)

Mix avocado, chopped celery, tomato, make open face sandwich
Total Carbs 14 grams or the approximate equivalent of 1 Diabetic exchange

Snack	<u>Strawberries,</u> sliced, fresh/frozen	1 cup (1 carb)
	Walnut halves, no salt	6 halves
	Water	16 fl oz

Total Carbs 13 grams or the approximate equivalent of 1 Diabetic exchange

Dinner	Tofu, extra firm, grilled, stir fry	3 oz
	<u>Asparagus, steamed/grilled</u>	11 spears (1/2 carb)
	Extra virgin olive oil	1 Tbsp
	<u>Brown rice</u>	1/3 c cooked (1 carb)

Add dill/salt free seasoning, drizzle olive oil, add black pepper
Total Carbs 20 grams or the approximate equivalent of 1.5 Diabetic exchanges

Snack	<u>Cantaloupe, diced</u>	1 cup (1 carb)
	Almond butter	2 tsp
	Water	16 fl oz

Total Carbs 13 grams or the approximate equivalent of 1Diabetic exchange

You Need to Know

Carbohydrates are underlined. Other foods may contain carbohydrates, but are not classified as carbs. Notice each meal or snack provides you with carbohydrate. Total carb grams plus diabetic exchange helps manage your total daily carb intake. Total carbs are distributed evenly throughout the day!

Jerrod P. Libonati, MS, RD

Day 4 Continued

Breakfast	Non-fat milk	4 fl oz (1/2 carb)
	Whole grain cereal	½ cup (1 carb)
	Banana, sliced	small (4") (1 carb)
	Flaxseeds	2 tsp
	Sliced almonds, unsalted	1 tsp
	Coffee	12 fl oz, 2 tsp nf milk
Snack	Whole wheat English muffin	½ each (1 carb)
	Benecol light/water	2 tsp/16 fl oz
	Coffee	8 fl oz, 2 tsp nf milk
Lunch	Loose leaf lettuce	2 leaves
	Tuna in water, low-sodium, Albacore	2 oz
	Tomato slices	3-4 slices
	Avocado	2 Tbsp
	Soybeans, steamed, no salt	½ cup (1 carb)

Mix avocado, chopped celery, tomato, make open face sandwich

Snack	Strawberries, sliced, fresh/frozen	1 cup (1 carb)
	Walnut halves, no salt/water	6 halves/16 fl oz
Dinner	Tofu, extra firm, grilled, stir fry	3 oz
	Asparagus, steamed/grilled	11 spears (1/2 carb)
	Extra virgin olive oil	1 Tbsp
	Brown rice	1/3 c cooked (1 carb)

Add dill/salt free seasoning, drizzle olive oil, add black pepper

Snack	Cantaloupe, diced	1 cup (1 carb)
	Almond butter/water	2 tsp/16 fl oz

Add Calories	1400 Calories	1500 Calories	1600 Calories	1700 Calories	1800 Calories
Breakfast		1 tsp seeds	1 tsp seeds	1 tsp seeds	4 fl oz milk 1/3 cup cereal 1 tsp seeds
Snack					
Lunch		1 oz tuna	1 oz tuna	1 oz tuna	1 oz tuna
Snack	½ c berries 3 w. halves	½ c berries 3 w. halves	½ c berries 3 w. halves	½ c berries 6 w. halves	½ c berries 6 w. halves
Dinner	1 tsp oil	2 oz tofu 1 tsp oil	2 oz tofu 1/3 c rice 2 tsp oil	2 oz tofu 1/3 c rice 2 tsp oil	2 oz tofu 1/3 c rice 2 tsp oil
Snack				1 tsp al. butter	1 tsp al. butter

Spacing Your Carbs

Breakfast	2.5	(more than 30, near 38 grams total carb)
Snack	1	(approximately 15 grams total carb)
Lunch	1	(approximately 15 grams total carb)
Snack	1	(approximately 15 grams total carb)
Dinner	1	(approximately 15 grams total carb)
Snack	1	(approximately 15 grams total carb)

Day 5

Breakfast	<u>Whole wheat toast</u>	1 slice (1 carb)
	Benecol light	2 tsp
	<u>Strawberries,</u> sliced, fresh/frozen	½ cup (1/2 carb)
	<u>Non-fat yogurt, plain/flavored</u>	6 oz (1 carb)
	Coffee	12 fl oz, 2 tsp nf milk

Total Carbs 35 grams or the approximate equivalent of 2 Diabetic exchanges

Snack	Low-fat/low-sodium cottage cheese	1/3 cup
	Water	16 fl oz
	Coffee	8 fl oz, 2 tsp nf milk

Total Carbs 2 grams or the approximate equivalent of 0 Diabetic exchanges

Lunch	<u>Rye bread</u>	1 slice (1 carb)
	Tuna in water, low-sodium, Albacore	3 oz
	<u>Tomato slices</u>	3-4 slices
	<u>Chopped celery</u>	1 Tbsp chopped
	Avocado	2 Tbsp
	<u>Orange</u>	1 medium (1 carb)

Mix avocado, chopped celery, open face sandwich, add tomato
Total Carbs 31 grams or the approximate equivalent of 2 Diabetic exchanges

Snack	<u>Non-fat yogurt, plain/flavored</u>	6 oz (1 carb)
	<u>Banana</u>	4" small (1 carb)
	Sesame seeds, unsalted	2 Tbsp
	Water	16 fl oz

Total Carbs 28 grams or the approximate equivalent of 2 Diabetic exchanges

Dinner	<u>Brown rice</u>	1/3 c cooked (1 carb)
	Halibut, grilled, broiled	3 oz
	Add herbs, salt free seasonings	
	Large Salad	
	<u>Spinach leaves, fresh, raw</u>	2 cups
	<u>Mixed greens</u>	2 cups
	<u>Tomato/cucumber slices</u>	2-3 slices each
	Salad dressing, lite	2 Tbsp
	Extra virgin olive oil	1 Tbsp
	<u>Broccoli,</u> steamed, no salt	1.5 cups (1 carb)

Add fresh lemon, drizzle olive oil, black pepper & salt free seasoning
Total Carbs 30 grams or the approximate equivalent of 2 Diabetic exchanges

Snack	<u>Cantaloupe,</u> diced	1 cup (1 carb)
	Water	16 fl oz

Total Carbs 13 grams or the approximate equivalent of 1 Diabetic exchange

You Need to Know

Carbohydrates are underlined. Other foods may contain carbohydrates, but are not classified as carbs. Notice each meal or snack provides you with carbohydrate. Total carb grams plus diabetic exchange helps manage your total daily carb intake. Total carbs are distributed evenly throughout the day!

Day 5 Continued

Breakfast	Whole wheat toast/Benecol light	1 slice (1 carb)/2 tsp
	Strawberries, sliced, fresh/frozen	½ cup (1/2 carb)
	Non-fat yogurt, plain/flavored	6 oz (1 carb)
	Coffee	12 fl oz, 2 tsp nf milk
Snack	Low-fat/low-sodium cottage cheese	1/3 cup
	Water	12 fl
	Coffee	8 fl oz, 2 tsp nf milk
Lunch	Rye bread	1 slice (1 carb)
	Tuna in water, low-sodium, Albacore	3 oz
	Tomato slices/Chopped celery	3-4 slices/1 Tbsp
	Avocado/Orange	2 Tbsp/ med. (1 carb)

Mix avocado, chopped celery, open face sandwich, add tomato

Snack	Non-fat yogurt, plain/flavored	6 oz (1 carb)
	Banana	4" small (1 carb)
	Sesame seeds, unsalted/water	2 Tbsp/16 fl oz
Dinner	Brown rice	1/3 c cooked (1 carb)
	Halibut, grilled, broiled (add salt free seasoning)	3 oz
	Large Salad	
	Spinach, fresh & mixed greens	2 cups each (1 carb)
	Tomato/cucumber slices	3-4 slices each
	Salad dressing, lite	2 Tbsp
	Extra virgin olive oil	1 Tbsp
	Broccoli, steamed, no salt	1.5 cups (1 carb)

Add fresh lemon to fish, olive oil on broccoli, add black pepper, add salt free seasoning

Snack	Cantaloupe, diced/water	1 c (1 carb)/16 fl oz

Add Calories	1400 Calories	1500 Calories	1600 Calories	1700 Calories	1800 Calories
Breakfast	2 tsp Benecol	2 tsp Benecol .5 c straw.	2 tsp Benecol 1 c straw.	2 tsp Benecol 1.5 c straw.	2 tsp Benecol 1.5 c straw.
Snack					
Lunch	2 tsp avocado	3 tsp avocado	2 tsp avocado	2 tsp avocado	2 tsp avocado
Snack	2 tsp seeds	3 tsp seeds		2 tsp seeds	3 tsp seeds
Dinner	1 oz fish 1 tsp oil	2 oz fish 1 tsp oil	3 oz fish 1 tsp oil	4 oz fish 1 tsp oil ½ c brocc	5 oz fish 1 tsp oil ½ c broccoli
Snack					½ c cantaloupe

Spacing Your Carbs

Breakfast	2	(approximately 30 grams total carb)
Snack	0	(less than 5 grams total carb)
Lunch	2	(approximately 30 grams total carb)
Snack	2	(approximately 30 grams total carb)
Dinner	2	(approximately 30 grams total carb)
Snack	1	(approximately 15 grams total carb)

Day 6

Breakfast	Blueberries, fresh/frozen	½ cup (1/2 carb)
	Cantaloupe, diced/cubed	1 cup (1 carb)
	Walnut halves, no salt	6 halves
	Coffee	12 fl oz, 2 tsp nf milk

Total Carbs 24 grams or the approximate equivalent of 2 Diabetic exchanges

Snack	Whole wheat English muffin	½ each (1 carb)
	Reduced fat peanut butter	2 tsp
	Non-fat milk	4 fl oz (1/2 carb)
	Coffee	8 fl oz, 2 tsp nf milk

Total Carbs 21 grams or the approximate equivalent of 1.5 Diabetic exchanges

Lunch	Chicken breast, white meat, no skin	3 oz (baked, broiled)
	Large Salad	
	Spinach, fresh & Salad greens	2 cups each (1 carb)
	Garbanzo beans, drained/rinsed	1/3 cup (1 carb)
	Tomato & cucumber slices	3-4 slices each
	Salad dressing, lite	2 Tbsp
	Water	16 fl oz

Mix greens, beans, tomato & cucumber w/dressing; add salt free seasoning & black pepper
Total Carbs 24 grams or the approximate equivalent of 2 Diabetic exchanges

Snack	Baby carrots	8 each (1/2 carb)
	Hummus, regular/flavored	2 Tbsp (1/2 carb)
	Water	16 fl oz

Total Carbs 12 grams or the approximate equivalent of 1 Diabetic exchange

Dinner	Halibut, baked, grilled, broiled	3 oz
	Broccoli, steamed, no salt	1.5 cups (1 carb)
	Benecol light	1 Tbsp
	Sweet potato, w/skin (tennis ball in size)	1 each (1 carb)
	Extra virgin olive oil	1 Tbsp

Add fresh lemon to fish, add Benecol to broccoli, add olive oil and black pepper to s. potato
Total Carbs 28 grams or the approximate equivalent of 2 Diabetic exchanges

Snack	Apple w/skin	1 small (1 carb)
	Water	16 fl oz

Total Carbs 17 grams or the approximate equivalent of 1 Diabetic exchange

You Need to Know

Notice your total carb intake was relatively stable throughout the day. You did not skip meals or snacks. Snacks provided enough carb to keep blood glucose consistent. Great job!

Day 6 Continued

Breakfast	Blueberries, fresh/frozen	½ cup (1/2 carb)
	Cantaloupe, diced/cubed/walnut halves	1 cup (1 carb)/6
	Coffee	12 fl oz, 2 tsp nf milk
Snack	Whole wheat English muffin	½ each (1 carb)
	Reduced fat peanut butter	2 tsp
	Non-fat milk	4 fl oz (1/2 carb)
	Coffee	8 fl oz, 2 tsp nf milk
Lunch	Chicken breast, white meat, no skin	3 oz (baked, broiled)
	Large Salad	
	Spinach, fresh & salad greens	2 cups each (1 carb)
	Garbanzo beans, drained/rinsed	1/3 cup (1 carb)
	Tomato & cucumber slices	3-4 slices each
	Salad dressing, lite/water	2 Tbsp/16 fl oz

Mix greens, beans, tomato, and cucumber into dressing; add salt free seasoning to chick breast

Snack	Baby carrots	8 each (1/2 carb)
	Hummus, regular/flavored	2 Tbsp (1/2 carb)
	Water	16 fl oz
Dinner	Halibut, baked, grilled, broiled	3 oz
	Broccoli, steamed, no salt	1.5 cups (1 carb)
	Benecol light	1 Tbsp
	Sweet potato, w/skin (tennis ball in size)	1 small (1 carb)
	Extra virgin olive oil	1 Tbsp

Add fresh lemon to fish, add Benecol to broccoli, add olive oil and black pepper to s. potato

Snack	Apple w/skin	1 medium (1 carb)
	Water	16 fl oz

Add Calories	1400 Calories	1500 Calories	1600 Calories	1700 Calories	1800 Calories
Breakfast	½ c berries	½ c berries 1 tsp Benecol	½ c berries 1 tsp Benecol	1 c berries 1 tsp Benecol 4 fl oz milk	1 c berries 2 tsp Benecol 4 fl oz milk
Snack					
Lunch	1/3 c beans	1/3 c beans	1/3 c beans	1/3 c beans	1/3 c beans
Snack					
Dinner		1 oz fish 1 tsp oil	2 oz fish 2 tsp oil	2 oz fish 2 tsp oil	3 oz fish 3 tsp oil
Snack					

Spacing Your Carbs

Breakfast	1.5	(more than 15, near 23 grams total carb)
Snack	1.5	(more than 15, near 23 grams total carb)
Lunch	2	(approximately 30 grams total carb)
Snack	1	(approximately 15 grams total carb)
Dinner	2	(approximately 30 grams total carb)
Snack	1	(approximately 15 grams total carb)

What State Do You Live In?

Day 7

Breakfast	<u>Non-fat milk</u>	4 fl oz (1/2 carb)
	<u>Whole grain cereal</u>	½ cup (1 carb)
	<u>Banana, sliced</u>	small (4") (1 carb)
	Flaxseeds	2 tsp
	Sliced almonds, unsalted	1 tsp
	Coffee	12 fl oz, 2 tsp nf milk

Total Carbs 40 grams or the approximate equivalent of 2.5 Diabetic exchanges

Snack	<u>Whole wheat English muffin</u>	½ each (1 carb)
	Benecol light	2 tsp
	Water	12 fl
	Coffee	8 fl oz, 2 tsp nf milk

Total Carbs 13 grams or the approximate equivalent of 1 Diabetic exchange

Lunch	<u>Loose leaf lettuce</u>	2 leaves
	Tuna in water, low-sodium, Albacore	2 oz
	<u>Tomato slices</u>	2-3 slices
	Avocado	2 Tbsp
	<u>Soybeans,</u> steamed, no salt	½ cup (1 carb)

Mix avocado, chopped celery, tomato, make open face sandwich
Total Carbs 14 grams or the approximate equivalent of 1Diabetic exchange

Snack	<u>Strawberries,</u> sliced, fresh/frozen	1 cup (1 carb)
	Walnut halves	6 halves
	Water	16 fl oz

Total Carbs 13 grams or the approximate equivalent of 1 Diabetic exchange

Dinner	Tofu, extra firm, grilled, stir fry	3 oz
	<u>Asparagus,</u> steamed/grilled	12 spears (1/2 carb)
	Extra virgin olive oil	1 Tbsp
	<u>Brown rice</u>	1/3 c cooked (1 carb)

Add dill/salt free seasoning, drizzle olive oil, add black pepper
Total Carbs 20 grams or the approximate equivalent of 1.5 Diabetic exchanges

Snack	<u>Cantaloupe,</u> diced	1 cup (1 carb)
	Almond butter	2 tsp

Total Carbs 13 grams or the approximate equivalent of 1Diabetic exchange

You Need to Know

Carbohydrates are underlined. Other foods may contain carbohydrates, but are not classified as carbs. Notice each meal or snack provides you with carbohydrate. Total carb grams plus diabetic exchange helps manage your total daily carb intake. Total carbs are distributed evenly throughout the day!

Jerrod P. Libonati, MS, RD

Day 7 Continued

Breakfast	Non-fat milk	4 fl oz (1/2 carb)
	Whole grain cereal	½ cup (1 carb)
	Banana, sliced	small (4") (1 carb)
	Flaxseeds	2 tsp
	Sliced almonds, unsalted	1 tsp
	Coffee	12 fl oz, 2 tsp nf milk
Snack	Whole wheat English muffin	½ each (1 carb)
	Benecol light	2 tsp
	Water	12 fl oz
	Coffee	8 fl oz, 2 tsp nf milk
Lunch	Loose leaf lettuce	2 leaves
	Tuna in water, low-sodium, Albacore	2 oz
	Tomato slices/Avocado	2-3 slices/2 Tbsp
	Soybeans, steamed, no salt	½ cup (1 carb)

Mix avocado, chopped celery, tomato; make open face sandwich

Snack	Strawberries, sliced, fresh/frozen	1 cup (1 carb)
	Walnut halves, no salt/water	6 halves/16 fl oz
Dinner	Tofu, extra firm, grilled, stir fry	3 oz
	Asparagus, steamed/grilled	12 spears (1/2 carb)
	Extra virgin olive oil	1 Tbsp
	Brown rice	1/3 c cooked (1 carb)

Add dill/salt free seasoning, drizzle olive, add black pepper

Snack	Cantaloupe, diced	1 cup (1 carb)
	Almond butter/water	2 tsp/16 fl oz

Add Calories	1400 Calories	1500 Calories	1600 Calories	1700 Calories	1800 Calories
Breakfast		1 tsp seeds	1 tsp seeds	1 tsp seeds	4 fl oz milk 1/3 c cereal 1 tsp seeds
Snack					
Lunch		1 oz tuna	1 oz tuna	1 oz tuna	1 oz tuna
Snack	½ c berries 3 w. halves	½ c berries 3 w. halves	½ c berries 3 w. halves	½ c berries 6 w. halves	½ c berries 6 w. halves
Dinner	1 tsp oil	2 oz tofu 1 tsp oil	2 oz tofu 1/3 c rice 2 tsp oil	2 oz tofu 1/3 c rice 2 tsp oil	2 oz tofu 1/3 c rice 2 tsp oil
Snack				1 tsp al. butter	1 tsp al. butter

Spacing Your Carbs

Breakfast	2.5	(more than 30 grams, near 37 grams total carb)
Snack	1	(approximately 15 grams total carb)
Lunch	1	(approximately 15 grams total carb)
Snack	1	(approximately 15 grams total carb)
Dinner	1.5	(more than 15, near 23 grams total carb)
Snack	1	(approximately 15 grams total carb)

Level 6 Weight Related Insulin Resistant Food Strategy

Level six is your most comprehensive weight related food strategy. It delivers all the nutrition and guidance you will need to reverse unhealthy blood glucose, cholesterol, triglycerides, and blood pressure. All foods used in designing this strategy come from your food portfolio. This food strategy is based on the guidelines provided by;

- The American Heart Association (AHA) and the National Cholesterol Education Program (NCEP) recommendations for managing blood cholesterol and triglycerides (lipids)

- The American Diabetic Association (ADA), a leading institution on diabetes and blood glucose management principals

- The National Heart, Lung and Blood Institute (NHLBI), a leading health agency on blood pressure and cardiovascular disease prevention

HIGHLIGHTS

Calories
- Plan listed is between 1,200 and 1,300 calories
- Five additional calorie levels have been added (1,400-1,800)
- Meal calories are distributed evenly throughout the day to help you lose weight and reverse insulin resistant related conditions
- Calories come from a variety of vitamin and mineral rich foods
- Snack calories are distributed evenly throughout the day to help control cravings and prevent overeating at meals

Carbohydrates
- Meals are carb controlled meaning they contain approximately the same amount of total carb grams, which helps maintain blood glucose
- Snacks are carb controlled meaning they contain approximately the same amount of total carb grams, which prevents overeating and curbs cravings
- All carbs used in this level are classified as "good" carbs meaning they provide you with sufficient nutrients and little added sugars

- All carbs are <u>underlined</u> to begin teaching you how to identify carb foods
- Meals and snacks that contain carbs are combined with protein and or fat to help slow the digestion and therefore the absorption of sugar (glucose) into the blood
- The Diabetic exchange system will help you count and control your carb intake.
- Average total carb percent per day = 48%
- Average carb grams per meal = 33 grams
- Average carb grams per snack = 12 grams

Protein
- Lean and very lean sources of animal protein are limited to help you control total fat, saturated fat, and dietary cholesterol
- Each day provides you with approximately 6-7 ounces of protein from animal sources including coldwater fish, which provide the heart healthy omega 3's
- Additional protein calories from plant based foods
- Average total protein percent per day = 19%

Fat
- Total Fat Average Per Day   32%
- Total Monounsaturated Fat Average/Day   17%
- Total Polyunsaturated Fat Average/Day   7%
- Total Saturated Fat Average/Day   4%
- Total Trans-fat Average/Day   <1%

Dietary Cholesterol
- Total Dietary Cholesterol Average/Day   54 milligrams

Spreads such as Benecol®, Benecol Light®, and Smart Balance® contain plant sterols, compounds that help lower total and LDL cholesterol are used in all examples

Additional Highlights
Each day provides you with the following nutrients used in lowering and managing blood pressure while providing artery health;

- Calcium Average   871 milligrams/day
- Potassium Average   2,300 milligrams/day

- Magnesium Average   306 milligrams/day
- Sodium Average   1,107 milligrams/day
- Fiber Average   30 grams/day

Good carbs, which include whole grains, fruit, and all vegetables, provide phytonutrients, compounds found in plants that fight chronic disease and promote cell protection. All seven days of examples are loaded with these nutrients that act in place of unnecessary supplementation.

Providing you with a variety of "good" carbs, healthy fats (mufas and pufas), and portion controlled lean proteins will collectively assist you in reversing your weight related insulin resistant state which may include, hypertriglyceridemia, hypertension, and low HDL cholesterol.

As a reminder, women should start with the plan listed, which is between 1,200-1,300 calories and men should start with the 1,500 calorie plan.

Jerrod P. Libonati, MS, RD

Level 6

Day 1

Breakfast
	Whole wheat toast/Benecol Light	1 slice (1 carb)/2 tsp
	Blueberries, fresh/frozen	½ cup (1/2 carb)
	Non-fat milk	4 fl oz (1/2 carb)
	Coffee	12 fl oz, 2 tsp nf milk

Total Carbs 39 grams or the approximate equivalent of 2 ½ Diabetic exchanges

Snack
	Banana (4")/Sesame seeds, unsalted	1 small/1 tbsp
	Coffee	8 fl oz, 2 tsp nf milk

Total Carbs 13 grams or the approximate equivalent of 1 Diabetic exchange

Lunch
	Spinach, raw	2 cups
	Tuna in water, low-sodium, Albacore	2 oz
	Bell peppers, sliced/chopped/Tomato slices	2 Tbsp/2-3 slices
	Kidney beans, drained/rinsed	1/3 cup (1 carb)
	Chopped celery/Avocado	1 tbsp chopped/2 tbsp
	Salad dressing, lite	2 Tbsp
	Cantaloupe, diced	1 cup (1 carb)
	Water	16 fl oz

Mix all ingredients into salad, add dressing and olive oil; cantaloupe as dessert
Total Carbs 26 grams or the approximate equivalent of 2 Diabetic exchanges

Snack
	Non-fat yogurt, plain/flavored	6 oz (1 carb)
	Whole grain cereal	½ cup (1 carb)
	Water	16 fl oz

Total Carbs 31 grams or the approximate equivalent of 2 Diabetic exchanges

Dinner
	Barley	1/3 c cooked (1 carb)
	Salmon, fresh/farmed (baked, grilled, broiled)	2 oz
	Broccoli, steamed, no salt	¾ cup (1 carb)
	Mushrooms, fresh/canned	1/3 cup
	Acorn squash, baked, w/skin	½ cup (1 carb)
	Olive oil	2 tsp

Add fresh lemon to fish, drizzle olive oil on broccoli & squash, add black pepper, salt free seasoning
Total Carbs 44 grams or the approximate equivalent of 3 Diabetic exchanges

Snack
	Sliced almonds, unsalted	2 tsp
	Water	16 fl oz

Total Carbs 0 grams or the approximate equivalent of 0 Diabetic exchanges

Carbohydrates are underlined. Carbs are evenly distributed throughout your day.
Total carb grams plus diabetic exchange helps manage your total daily carb intake.

Total Fat	Sat Fat	Mono Fat	Cholesterol	Calcium	Magnesium	Potassium	Sodium	Fiber
45	6	22	58	741	361	3,104	999	39

Fats and fiber measured in grams (g); cholesterol and others in milligrams (mg)

Day 1 Continued

Breakfast	Whole wheat toast	1 slice (1 carb)
	Benecol light	2 tsp
	Blueberries, fresh/frozen	½ cup (1/2 carb)
	Non-fat milk	4 fl oz (1/2 carb)
	Coffee	12 fl oz, 2 tsp nf milk
Snack	Banana (4")/Sesame seeds, unsalted	1 small/1 tbsp
	Coffee	8 fl oz, 2 tsp nf milk
Lunch	Spinach, raw	2 cups
	Tuna in water, low-sodium, Albacore	2 oz
	Bell peppers, sliced/chopped, tomato slices	2 tbsp, 2-3 slices
	Kidney beans, drained/rinsed	1/3 cup (1 carb)
	Chopped celery/Avocado	1 Tbsp /2 Tbsp
	Salad dressing, lite	2 Tbsp
	Cantaloupe, diced/cubed	1 cup (1 carb)
	Water	16 fl oz

Mix all ingredients into salad, add dressing and olive oil; cantaloupe as dessert

Snack	Non-fat yogurt, plain/flavored	6 oz (1 carb)
	Whole grain cereal	½ cup (1 carb)
	Water	16 fl oz
Dinner	Barley	1/3 c cooked (1 carb)
	Salmon, baked, grilled	2 oz
	Broccoli, steamed, no salt	¾ cup (1 carb)
	Mushrooms, fresh/canned	1/3 cup
	Acorn squash, baked, w/skin	½ cup (1 carb)
	Olive oil	2 tsp
	Water	16 fl oz

Add fresh lemon to fish, drizzle olive oil on broccoli & squash, add black pepper, salt free seasoning

Snack	Sliced almonds, unsalted	2 tsp
	Water	16 fl oz

Add Calories	1400 Calories	1500 Calories	1600 Calories	1700 Calories	1800 Calories
Breakfast	1 tsp Benecol	1 tsp Benecol	1 tsp Benecol	1 tsp Benecol ½ c berries	1 tsp Benecol ½ c berries
Snack		1 Tbsp seeds	1 Tbsp seeds	1 Tbsp seeds	1 Tbsp seeds
Lunch			1 c spinach 2 tsp oil	1 c spinach 2 tsp oil	1 c spinach 2 tsp oil
Snack					
Dinner	1 oz salmon 1 tsp oil	1 oz salmon 2 tsp oil	1 oz salmon 2 tsp oil	1 oz salmon ½ c broccoli 2 tsp oil	2 oz salmon ½ c broccoli 3 tsp oil
Snack				2 tsp almonds	2 tsp almonds

Jerrod P. Libonati, MS, RD

Day 2

Breakfast	<u>Whole grain cereal</u>	½ cup (1 carb)
	Sliced almonds, unsalted	2 tsp
	<u>Strawberries</u>, sliced, fresh/frozen	½ cup (1/2 carb)
	<u>Non-fat milk</u>	4 fl. oz (1/2 carb)
	Coffee	12 fl oz, 2 tsp nf milk

Total Carbs 32 grams or the approximate equivalent of 2 Diabetic exchanges

Snack	<u>Rye bread</u>	1 slice (1 carb)
	Benecol Light	2 tsp
	Coffee	8 fl oz, 2 tsp nf milk

Total Carbs 12 grams or the approximate equivalent of 1 Diabetic exchange

Lunch	Turkey breast slices, low-sodium	2 oz
	Fat free mayo	2 tsp
	<u>Tomato slices</u>	2-3 slices
	<u>Whole wheat tortilla (6")</u>	1 small (1 carb)
	<u>Loose leaf lettuce</u>	2 leaves
	Avocado	2 Tbsp
	Salad dressing, lite	1 Tbsp
	<u>Orange</u>	1 small (1 carb)
	Water	16 fl oz

Make tortilla sandwich; orange as dessert
Total Carbs 40 grams or the approximate equivalent of 2 ½ Diabetic exchanges

Snack	<u>Non-fat yogurt, plain/flavored</u>	6 oz (1 carb)
	Sesame seeds, unsalted	2 Tbsp
	Flaxseeds	1 Tbsp
	Water	16 fl oz

Total Carbs 18 grams or the approximate equivalent of 1 Diabetic exchange

Dinner	<u>S. potato</u>, baked w/ skin (tennis ball size)	1 (1 carb)
	Chick breast, white meat, no skin, baked/broiled	2 oz
	<u>Spinach</u>, stir fry, no salt, cooked	1 cup (1/2 carb)
	Olive oil	2 tsp

Drizzle olive oil on potato and spinach, add garlic, onion, black pepper, salt free seasoning
Total Carbs 26 grams or the approximate equivalent of 2 Diabetic exchanges

Snack	Almond butter	2 tsp
	<u>Non-fat milk</u>	4 fl oz (1/2 carb)

Total Carbs 7 grams or the approximate equivalent of 1/2 Diabetic exchange

Carbohydrates are underlined. Carbs are evenly distributed throughout your day.
Total carb grams plus diabetic exchange helps you manage your total daily carb intake.

Total Fat	Sat Fat	Mono Fat	Cholesterol	Calcium	Magnesium	Potassium	Sodium	Fiber
46	5	23	57	1,085	475	2,640	976	29

Fats and fiber measured in grams (g); cholesterol and others in milligrams (mg)

Day 2 Continued

Breakfast	Whole grain cereal	½ cup (1 carb)
	Sliced almonds, unsalted	2 tsp
	Strawberries, sliced, fresh/frozen	½ cup (1/2 carb)
	Non-fat milk	4 fl oz (1/2 carb)
	Coffee	12 fl oz, 2 tsp nf milk
Snack	Rye bread	1 slice (1 carb)
	Benecol light	2 tsp
	Coffee	8 fl oz, 2 tsp nf milk
Lunch	Turkey breast slices, low-sodium	2 oz
	Fat free mayo	2 tsp
	Tomato slices	2-3 slices
	Whole wheat tortilla (6")	1 small (1 carb)
	Loose leaf lettuce	2 leaves
	Avocado	2 Tbsp
	Salad dressing, lite	1 Tbsp
	Orange	1 small (1 carb)
	Water	16 fl oz

Make tortilla sandwich; orange as dessert

Snack	Non-fat yogurt, plain/flavored	6 oz (1 carb)
	Sesame seeds, unsalted	2 Tbsp
	Flaxseeds	1 Tbsp
	Water	16 fl oz
Dinner	S. potato, baked w/ skin (tennis ball size)	1 (1 carb)
	Chick breast, white meat, no skin, bakd/broil	2 oz
	Spinach, stir fry, no salt, cooked	1 cup
	Olive oil	2 tsp
	Water	16 fl oz

Drizzle olive oil on potato and spinach, add garlic, onion, black pepper, salt free seasoning

Snack	Almond butter	2 tsp
	Non-fat milk	4 fl oz (1/2 carb)

Add Calories	1400 Calories	1500 Calories	1600 Calories	1700 Calories	1800 Calories
Breakfast	½ c berries	1 c berries	2 tsp almonds 1 c berries	2 tsp almonds 1 c berries	3 tsp almonds 1 c berries
Snack		1 tsp Benecol	1 tsp Benecol	1 tsp Benecol	2 tsp Benecol
Lunch		1 oz tuna	1 oz tuna	2 oz tuna	2 oz tuna
Snack					
Dinner	1 tsp oil	2 tsp oil	1 oz chicken 2 tsp oil	2 oz chicken 2 tsp oil	3 oz chicken 3 tsp oil
Snack	1 tsp al butter	1 tsp al butter	2 tsp al butter	2 tsp al butter 4 fl oz milk	2 tsp al butter 4 fl oz milk

Jerrod P. Libonati, MS, RD

Day 3

Breakfast		
	Oatmeal, cooked	½ cup (1 carb)
	Flaxseeds	1 Tbsp
	Blueberries, fresh	½ cup (1/2 carb)
	Non-fat milk	4 fl. oz (1/2 carb)
	Coffee	12 f oz, 2 tsp nf milk

Total Carbs 31 grams or the approximate equivalent of 2 Diabetic exchanges

Snack		
	Cantaloupe, diced/cubed	1 cup (1 carb)
	Walnuts, chopped	2 Tbsp
	Coffee	8 fl oz, 2 tsp nf milk

Total Carbs 13 grams or the approximate equivalent of 1 Diabetic exchange

Lunch		
	Chicken breast, white meat, shredded	2 oz
	Avocado	1 Tbsp
	Tomato slices	2-3 slices
	Whole wheat tortilla (6")	1 small (1 carb)
	Loose leaf lettuce	1 leaf
	Spinach, raw	½ cup
	Cantaloupe	1 cup (1 carb)
	Water	16 fl oz

Make tortilla sandwich; cantaloupe as dessert
Total Carbs 37 grams or the approximate equivalent of 2.5 Diabetic exchanges

Snack		
	Non-fat yogurt, plain/flavored	6 oz (1 carb)
	Sesame seeds, unsalted/flaxseeds	1 Tbsp/1 Tbsp
	Water	12 fl oz

Total Carbs 17 grams or the approximate equivalent of 1 Diabetic exchange

Dinner		
	Broccoli, steamed, no salt	¾ cup (1/2 carb)
	Whole wheat pasta noodles, cooked	½ cup (1 carb)
	Marinara sauce, low sodium	1/3 cup
	Kidney beans, rinsed	1/3 cup (1 carb)
	Olive oil	2 tsp
	Water	16 fl oz

Mix beans w/pasta and sauce; drizzle olive oil on broccoli, add garlic, black pepper, salt free seasoning
Total Carbs 47 grams or the approximate equivalent of 3 Diabetic exchanges

Snack		
	Almond butter	2 tsp
	Non-fat yogurt	6 oz (1 carb)

Total Carbs 17 grams or the approximate equivalent of 1 Diabetic exchange

Carbohydrates are underlined. Carbs are evenly distributed throughout your day.
Total carb grams plus diabetic exchange helps manage your total daily carb intake.

Total Fat	Sat Fat	Mono Fat	Cholesterol	Calcium	Magnesium	Potassium	Sodium	Fiber
43	5	17	42	713	264	2,000	684	32

Fats and fiber measured in grams (g); cholesterol and others in milligrams (mg)

What State Do You Live In?

Day 3 Continued

Breakfast	Oatmeal, cooked	½ cup (1 carb)
	Flaxseeds	1 Tbsp
	Blueberries, fresh	½ cup (1/2 carb)
	Non-fat milk	4 fl. oz (1/2 carb)
	Coffee	12 fl oz, 2 tsp nf milk
Snack	Cantaloupe	1 cup (1 carb)
	Walnuts, chopped	2 Tbsp
	Coffee	8 fl oz, 2 tsp nf milk
Lunch	Chicken breast, white meat, shredded	2 oz
	Avocado	1 Tbsp
	Tomato slices	2-3 slices
	Whole wheat tortilla (6")	1 small (1 carb)
	Loose leaf lettuce	1 leaf
	Spinach, raw	½ cup
	Cantaloupe	1 cup (1 carb)
	Water	12 fl oz

Make tortilla sandwich; cantaloupe as dessert

Snack	Non-fat yogurt, plain/flavored	6 oz (1 carb)
	Sesame seeds, unsalted/flaxseeds	1 Tbsp/1 Tbsp
	Water	12 fl oz
Dinner	Broccoli, steamed, no salt	¾ cup (1/2 carb)
	Whole wheat pasta noodles, cooked	½ cup (1 carb)
	Marinara sauce, low sodium	1/3 cup
	Kidney beans, rinsed	1/3 cup (1 carb)
	Olive oil	2 tsp
	Water	12 fl oz

Mix beans w/pasta and sauce; drizzle olive oil on broccoli, add garlic, black pepper, salt free seasoning

Snack	Almond butter	2 tsp
	Non-fat yogurt, flavored/plain	6 oz (1 carb)

Add Calories	1400 Calories	1500 Calories	1600 Calories	1700 Calories	1800 Calories
Breakfast			½ c berries	1 c berries	1 c berries
Snack	1 Tbsp walnuts	1 Tbsp walnuts	1 Tbsp walnuts	1 Tbsp walnuts	1 Tbsp walnuts
Lunch			1 oz chicken	2 oz chicken	2 oz chicken
Snack			2 tsp flaxseed		1 tsp flaxseed
Dinner	1 tsp olive oil	½ c broccoli 2 tsp olive oil	½ c broccoli 2 tsp olive oil	½ c broccoli 3 tsp olive oil	½ c pasta ½ c broccoli 3 tsp olive oil
Snack		1 tsp al. butter	1 tsp al. butter	1 tsp al. butter	1 tsp al. butter

Jerrod P. Libonati, MS, RD

Day 4

Breakfast		
	Rye toast	1 slice (1 carb)
	Benecol Light	1 Tbsp
	Kiwi, fresh	4-5 slices (1/2 carb)
	Non-fat milk	4 fl. oz (1/2 carb)
	Coffee	12 fl oz, 2 tsp nf milk

Total Carbs 26 grams or the approximate equivalent of 2 Diabetic exchanges

Snack		
	Non-fat yogurt, flavored/plain	6 oz (1 carb)
	Flaxseeds	2 Tbsp
	Coffee	8 fl oz, 2 tsp nf milk

Total Carbs 17 grams or the approximate equivalent of 1 Diabetic exchange

Lunch		
	Large Salad	
	Spinach, raw	2 cups (1/2 carb)
	Salad greens	2 cups (1/2 carb)
	Tomato & cucumber slices	3-4 slices each
	Sesame seeds, unsalted	1 Tbsp
	Kidney beans, rinsed	1/3 cup (1 carb)
	Extra virgin olive oil	2 tsp
	Salad dressing, lite	2 Tbsp

Mix all ingredients
Total Carbs 37 grams or the approximate equivalent of 2.5 Diabetic exchanges

Snack		
	Non-fat yogurt, plain/flavored	6 oz (1 carb)
	Sesame seeds, unsalted	1 Tbsp
	Flaxseeds	1 Tbsp
	Water	12 fl oz

Total Carbs 17 grams or the approximate equivalent of 1 Diabetic exchange

Dinner		
	Salmon, fresh/farmed, (baked, grilled, broiled)	2 oz
	Broccoli, steamed, no salt	1.5 cups (1 carb)
	Brown rice, cooked	1/3 cup (1 carb)
	Olive oil	2 tsp
	Water	12 fl oz

Mix beans w/pasta & sauce; drizzle oil on broccoli, add garlic, black pepper, salt free seasoning
Total Carbs 30 grams or the approximate equivalent of 2 Diabetic exchanges

Snack		
	Almond butter	2 tsp
	Non-fat milk	4 fl oz (1/2 carb)

Total Carbs 7 grams or the approximate equivalent of ½ Diabetic exchange

Carbohydrates are underlined. Carbs are evenly distributed throughout your day.
Total carb grams plus diabetic exchange helps manage your total daily carb intake.

Total Fat	Sat Fat	Mono Fat	Cholesterol	Calcium	Magnesium	Potassium	Sodium	Fiber
58	7	29	46	892	228	1,786	1,114	31

Fats and fiber measured in grams (g); cholesterol and others in milligrams (mg)

Day 4 Continued

Breakfast	Rye toast	1 slice (1 carb)
	Benecol Light	1 Tbsp
	Kiwi, fresh	4-5 slices (1/2 carb)
	Non-fat milk	4 fl oz (1/2 carb)
	Coffee	12 fl oz, 2 tsp nf milk
Snack	Non-fat yogurt, flavored/plain	6 oz (1 carb)
	Flaxseeds	2 Tbsp
	Coffee	8 fl oz, 2 tsp nf milk
Lunch	Large Salad	
	Spinach, raw	2 cups (1/2 carb)
	Salad greens	2 cups (1/2 carb)
	Tomato & cucumber slices	3-4 slices each
	Sesame seeds, unsalted	1 Tbsp
	Kidney beans, rinsed	1/3 cup (1 carb)
	Extra virgin olive oil	2 tsp
	Salad dressing, lite	2 Tbsp

Mix all ingredients

Snack	Non-fat yogurt, plain/flavored	6 oz (1 carb)
	Sesame seeds, unsalted	1 Tbsp
	Flaxseeds	1 Tbsp
	Water	12 fl oz
Dinner	Salmon, fresh/farmed, (baked, grilled, broiled)	2 oz
Broccoli, steamed, no salt		1.5 cups (1 carb)
	Brown rice, cooked	1/3 cup (1 carb)
	Olive oil	2 tsp
	Water	12 fl oz

Mix beans w/pasta & sauce; drizzle oil on broccoli, add garlic, black pepper, salt free seasoning

Snack	Almond butter	2 tsp
	Non-fat milk	4 fl oz (1/2 carb)

Add Calories	1400 Calories	1500 Calories	1600 Calories	1700 Calories	1800 Calories
Breakfast		2 slices kiwi	4 slices kiwi 4 fl oz milk	4 slices kiwi 4 fl oz milk	4 slices kiwi 4 fl oz milk
Snack					
Lunch	1 tsp oil	1 tsp oil	2 tsp oil	2 tsp oil	2 tsp oil
Snack	1 tsp seeds	1 tsp seeds	1 tsp seeds	1 tsp seeds	1 tsp seeds
Dinner	1 tsp oil	1 oz fish 1 tsp oil	1 oz fish 1 tsp oil	3 oz fish 1 tsp oil	4 oz fish 1 tsp oil
Snack		1 tsp al butter	1 tsp al butter		4 fl oz milk

Jerrod P. Libonati, MS, RD

Day 5

Breakfast		
	Blueberries, fresh	½ cup (1/2 carb)
	Strawberries, fresh	½ c sliced (1/2 carb)
	Non-fat yogurt	6 oz (1 carb)
	Flaxseeds	2 Tbsp
	Coffee	12 fl oz, 2 tsp nf milk

Total Carbs 34 grams or the approximate equivalent of 2 Diabetic exchanges

Snack		
	Whole wheat English muffin	½ (1 carb)
	Almond butter	2 tsp
	Non-fat milk	4 fl oz (1/2 carb)
	Coffee	8 fl oz, 2 tsp nf milk

Total Carbs 20 grams or the approximate equivalent of 1 Diabetic exchange

Lunch		
	Large Salad	
	Spinach, raw	2 cups (1/2 carb)
	Salad greens	2 cups (1/2 carb)
	Tomato slices	3-4 pieces
	Cucumber slices	3-4 pieces
	Sesame seeds, unsalted	1 Tbsp
	Tuna, low sodium, Albacore	2 oz
	Extra virgin olive oil	2 tsp
	Salad dressing, lite	2 Tbsp
	Water	12 fl oz

Mix all ingredients
Total Carbs 15 grams or the approximate equivalent of 1 Diabetic exchange

Snack		
	Non-fat yogurt, plain/flavored	6 oz (1 carb)
	Flaxseeds	1 Tbsp
	Water	12 fl oz

Total Carbs 17 grams or the approximate equivalent of 1 Diabetic exchange

Dinner		
	Tofu, extra firm, grilled, stir fry	3 oz
	Asparagus, steamed/grilled	11 spears (1/2 carb)
	Extra virgin olive oil	1 Tbsp
	Brown rice	1/3 c cooked (1 carb)

Add dill/salt free seasoning to tofu, drizzle olive oil on asparagus, add black pepper, salt free seasoning
Total Carbs 20 grams or the approximate equivalent of 1.5 Diabetic exchanges

Snack		
	Almond butter	2 tsp
	Non-fat milk	4 fl oz (1/2 carb)

Total Carbs 7 grams or the approximate equivalent of ½ Diabetic exchange

Carbohydrates are underlined. Carbs are evenly distributed throughout your day.
Total carb grams plus diabetic exchange helps manage your total daily carb intake.

Total Fat	Sat Fat	Mono Fat	Cholesterol	Calcium	Magnesium	Potassium	Sodium	Fiber
47	5	23	28	1,017	172	1,361	1,089	23

Fats and fiber measured in grams (g); cholesterol and others in milligrams (mg)

Day 5 Continued

Breakfast	Blueberries, fresh	½ cup (1/2 carb)
	Strawberries, fresh	½ c sliced (1/2 carb)
	Non-fat yogurt	6 oz (1 carb)
	Flaxseeds	2 Tbsp
	Coffee	12 fl oz, 2 tsp nf milk
Snack	Whole wheat English muffin	½ (1 carb)
	Almond butter	2 tsp
	Non-fat milk	4 fl oz (1/2 carb)
	Coffee	8 fl oz, 2 tsp nf milk
Lunch	Large Salad	
	Spinach, raw	2 cups (1/2 carb)
	Salad greens	2 cups (1/2 carb)
	Tomato slices	3-4 pieces
	Cucumber slices	3-4 pieces
	Sesame seeds, unsalted	1 Tbsp
	Tuna, low sodium, Albacore	2 oz
	Extra virgin olive oil	2 tsp
	Salad dressing, lite	2 Tbsp
	Water	12 fl oz

Mix all ingredients

Snack	Non-fat yogurt, plain/flavored	6 oz (1 carb)
	Flaxseeds	1 Tbsp
	Water	12 fl oz
Dinner	Tofu, extra firm, grilled, stir fry	3 oz
	Asparagus, steamed/grilled	11 spears (1/2 carb)
	Extra virgin olive oil	1 Tbsp
	Brown rice	1/3 c cooked (1 carb)

Add dill/salt free seasoning to tofu, drizzle olive oil on asparagus, add black pepper, salt free seasoning

Snack	Almond butter	2 tsp
	Non-fat milk	4 fl oz (1/2 carb)

Add Calories	1400 Calories	1500 Calories	1600 Calories	1700 Calories	1800 Calories
Breakfast	1 c berries	1 c berries	1.5 c berries	1.5 c berries	1.5 c berries
Snack			4 fl oz milk	4 fl oz milk	4 fl oz milk
Lunch			1 oz tuna	1 oz tuna	1 oz tuna
Snack					
Dinner	5 s. asparagus	5 s. asparagus 1 tsp oil 1/3 c rice	5 s. asparagus 1 tsp oil 1/3 c rice	2 oz tofu 5 s. asparagus 2 tsp oil 1/3 c rice	3 oz tofu 11 s. asparagus 2 tsp oil 1/3 c rice
Snack	4 fl oz milk	4 fl oz milk	4 fl oz milk	4 fl oz milk	1 tsp a butter 4 fl oz milk

Day 6

Breakfast	<u>Whole grain cereal</u>	½ cup (1 carb)
	Sliced almonds, unsalted	2 tsp
	<u>Blueberries</u>, fresh/frozen	½ cup (1/2 carb)
	<u>Non-fat milk</u>	4 fl oz (1/2 carb)
	Coffee	12 fl oz, 2 tsp nf milk

Total Carbs 37 grams or the approximate equivalent of 2.5 Diabetic exchanges

Snack	<u>Cantaloupe</u>, diced/cubed	1 cup (1 carb)
	Sliced almonds, unsalted	2 tsp
	Coffee	8 fl oz, 2 tsp nf milk

Total Carbs 13 grams or the approximate equivalent of 1 Diabetic exchange

Lunch	Turkey breast slices, low-sodium	2 oz
	Fat free mayo	2 tsp
	<u>Tomato slices</u>	2-3 slices
	<u>Whole wheat tortilla (6")</u>	1 small (1 carb)
	<u>Loose leaf lettuce</u>	2 leaves
	Avocado	2 Tbsp
	Salad dressing, lite	2 Tbsp
	<u>Orange</u>	1 small (1 carb)
	Water	12 fl oz

Make tortilla sandwich; orange as dessert
Total Carbs 40 grams or the approximate equivalent of 2.5 Diabetic exchanges

Snack	<u>Non-fat yogurt, plain/flavored</u>	6 oz (1 carb)
	Flaxseeds	1 Tbsp
	Water	12 fl oz

Total Carbs 17 grams or the approximate equivalent of 1 Diabetic exchange

Dinner	<u>S. potato</u>, baked w/ skin (tennis ball size)	1 (1 carb)
	Chick breast, white meat, no skin, baked/broiled	2 oz
	<u>Spinach</u>, stir fry, no salt, cooked	1 cup
	Olive oil	1 Tbsp

Drizzle olive oil on potato and spinach, add garlic, onion, black pepper, salt free seasoning
Total Carbs 26 grams or the approximate equivalent of 2 Diabetic exchanges

Snack	Almond butter	2 tsp
	<u>Non-fat milk</u>	4 fl oz (1/2 carb)

Total Carbs 7 grams or the approximate equivalent of 1/2 Diabetic exchange

Carbohydrates are underlined. Carbs are evenly distributed throughout your day. Total carb grams plus diabetic exchange helps manage your total daily carb intake.

Total Fat	Sat Fat	Mono Fat	Cholesterol	Calcium	Magnesium	Potassium	Sodium	Fiber
40	4	21	66	1,039	401	3,157	1,649	27

Fats and fiber measured in grams (g); cholesterol and others in milligrams (mg)

Day 6 Continued

Breakfast	Whole grain cereal	½ cup (1 carb)
	Sliced almonds, unsalted	2 tsp
	Blueberries, fresh, frozen	½ cup (1/2 carb)
	Non-fat milk	4 fl oz (1/2 carb)
	Coffee	12 fl oz, 2 tsp nf milk
Snack	Cantaloupe, diced/cubed	1 cup (1 carb)
	Sliced almonds, unsalted	2 tsp
	Coffee	8 fl oz, 2 tsp nf milk
Lunch	Turkey breast slices, low-sodium	2 oz
	Fat free mayo	2 tsp
	Tomato slices	2-3 slices
	Whole wheat tortilla (6")	1 small (1 carb)
	Loose leaf lettuce	2 leaves
	Avocado	2 Tbsp
	Salad dressing, lite	2 Tbsp
	Orange	1 small (1 carb)
	Water	12 fl oz

Make tortilla sandwich; orange as dessert

Snack	Non-fat yogurt, plain/flavored	6 oz (1 carb)
	Flaxseeds	1 Tbsp
	Water	12 fl oz
Dinner	S. potato, baked w/ skin (tennis ball size)	1 (1 carb)
	Chick breast/white meat/no skin/baked/broiled	2 oz
	Spinach, stir fry, no salt, cooked	1 cup
	Olive oil	1 Tbsp

Drizzle olive oil on potato and spinach, add garlic, onion, black pepper, salt free seasoning

Snack	Almond butter	2 tsp
	Non-fat milk	4 fl oz (1/2 carb)

Add Calories	1400 Calories	1500 Calories	1600 Calories	1700 Calories	1800 Calories
Breakfast	½ c berries	½ c cereal ½ c berries	½ c cereal 1 tsp almonds ½ c berries	½ c cereal 2 tsp almonds 1 c berries	1 c cereal 2 tsp almonds 1 c berries
Snack			1 tsp almonds	1 tsp almonds	1 tsp almonds
Lunch					
Snack					
Dinner			1 oz chicken 1 tsp oil	2 oz chicken 1 tsp oil	2 oz chicken 1 tsp oil
Snack	1 tsp al butter 4 fl oz milk	1 tsp al butter 4 fl oz milk	1 tsp al butter 4 fl oz milk	1 tsp al butter 4 fl oz milk	1 tsp al butter 4 fl oz milk

Jerrod P. Libonati, MS, RD

Day 7

Breakfast
Oatmeal, cooked	½ cup (1 carb)
Flaxseeds	1 Tbsp
Blueberries, fresh/frozen	½ cup (1/2 carb)
Non-fat milk	4 fl oz (1/2 carb)
Coffee	12 fl oz, 2 tsp nf milk

Total Carbs 31 grams or the approximate equivalent of 2 Diabetic exchanges

Snack
Strawberries, sliced, fresh/frozen	1 cup (1 carb)
Walnuts, chopped	2 Tbsp
Coffee	8 fl oz, 2 tsp nf milk

Total Carbs 13 grams or the approximate equivalent of 1 Diabetic exchange

Lunch
Chicken breast, white meat, shredded	2 oz
Avocado	1 Tbsp
Tomato slices	2-3 slices
Whole wheat tortilla (6")	1 small (1 carb)
Loose leaf lettuce	1 leaf
Spinach, raw	½ cup
Orange	1 small (1 carb)
Water	12 fl oz

Make tortilla sandwich; orange as dessert
Total Carbs 38 grams or the approximate equivalent of 2.5 Diabetic exchanges

Snack
Non-fat yogurt, plain/flavored	6 oz (1 carb)
Sesame seeds, unsalted	1 Tbsp
Flaxseeds	1 Tbsp
Water	12 fl oz

Total Carbs 17 grams or the approximate equivalent of 1 Diabetic exchange

Dinner
Broccoli, steamed, no salt	1.5 cups (1 carb)
Whole wheat pasta noodles, cooked	½ cup (1 carb)
Marinara sauce, low sodium	1/3 cup
Ground turkey, lean	2 oz
Olive oil	2 tsp
Water	12 fl oz

Mix turkey w/pasta/sauce; drizzle oil on broccoli, add garlic, black pepper, salt free seasoning
Total Carbs 37 grams or the approximate equivalent of 2.5 Diabetic exchanges

Snack
Sliced almonds, unsalted	2 tsp
Non-fat yogurt	6 oz (1 carb)

Total Carbs 17 grams or the approximate equivalent of 1 Diabetic exchange

Carbohydrates are underlined. Carbs are evenly distributed throughout your day.
Total carb grams plus diabetic exchange helps manage your total daily carb intake.

Total Fat	Sat Fat	Mono Fat	Cholesterol	Calcium	Magnesium	Potassium	Sodium	Fiber
45	5	16	83	611	246	2,030	608	32

Fats and fiber measured in grams (g); cholesterol and others in milligrams (mg)

What State Do You Live In?

Day 7 Continued

Breakfast	Oatmeal, cooked/Flaxseeds	½ cup (1 carb)/Tbsp
	Blueberries, fresh/frozen	½ cup (1/2 carb)
	Non-fat milk	4 fl oz (1/2 carb)
	Coffee	12 fl oz, 2 tsp nf milk
Snack	Strawberries, sliced, fresh/frozen	1 cup (1 carb)
	Walnuts, chopped	2 Tbsp
	Coffee	8 fl oz, 2 tsp nf milk
Lunch	Chicken breast, white meat, shredded	2 oz
	Avocado	1 Tbsp
	Tomato slices	2-3 slices
	Whole wheat tortilla (6")	1 small (1 carb)
	Loose leaf lettuce	1 leaf
	Spinach, raw	½ cup
	Orange	1 small (1 carb)
	Water	12 fl oz

Make tortilla sandwich; orange as dessert

Snack	Non-fat yogurt, plain/flavored	6 oz (1 carb)
	Sesame seeds, unsalted	1 Tbsp
	Flaxseeds	1 Tbsp
	Water	12 fl oz
Dinner	Broccoli, steamed, no salt	1.5 cups (1 carb)
	Whole wheat pasta noodles, cooked	½ cup (1 carb)
	Marinara sauce, low sodium	1/3 cup
	Ground turkey, lean	2 oz
	Olive oil	2 tsp
	Water	12 fl oz

Mix turkey w/pasta/sauce; oil on broccoli, add garlic, black pepper, salt free seasoning

Snack	Sliced almonds, unsalted	2 tsp
	Non-fat yogurt	6 oz (1 carb)

Add Calories	1400 Calories	1500 Calories	1600 Calories	1700 Calories	1800 Calories
Breakfast	½ c berries	½ c berries	1 c berries	½ c oatmeal 1 c berries 2 fl oz milk	½ c oatmeal 1 c berries 4 fl oz milk
Snack		1 Tbsp walnuts	1 Tbsp walnuts	1 Tbsp walnuts	1 Tbsp walnuts
Lunch		1 Tbsp avocado	1 Tbsp avocado	1 Tbsp avocado	1 Tbsp avocado
Snack					1 tbsp sesame
Dinner	1 tsp oil	1 oz turkey 1 tsp oil	½ c broccoli 1 oz turkey 2 tsp oil	½ c broccoli 1 oz turkey 2 tsp oil	½ c broccoli 2 oz turkey 2 tsp oil
Snack	1 tsp almonds	1 tsp almonds	1 tsp almonds	1 tsp almonds	1 tsp almonds

Selected References

Section I   The Healthy State

Barter, P.J. (2002) Hugh sinclair lecture: The regulation and remodeling of HDL by plasma factors. Atherosclerosis Supplements. 3:39-47.

Cooper, A.D. (1997) Hepatic uptake of chyomicron remnants. J Lipid Res. 38:2173-2192.

Curtiss, L.K., Valenta, D.T., Hime, N.J., and Rye, K.A. (2006) What is so special about apolipoprotein A1 in reverse cholesterol transport? Arterioscler Thromb Vasc Biol. 26:12-19.

Eckel, R.H., Yost, T.J., and Jensen, D.R. (1995) Alterations in lipoprotein lipase in insulin resistance. Inter J Obes Relat Met Disord. May 19 suppl. 1:S16-21.

Eisenberg, S. (1983) Lipoproteins and lipoprotein metabolism. Klin Wochenschr. 61:119-132.

Fielding, C. J., and Fielding, P.E. (1995) Molecular physiology of reverse cholesterol transport. J. Lipid Res. 36:211-228.

Ginsberg, H.N. (1998) Lipoprotein Physiology. Lipoprotein Disorders. 27:503-518.

Gupta, A.K., Ross, E.A., Myers, J.N., and Kashyap, M.L. (1993) Increased reverse cholesterol transport in athletes. 42:684-690.

Klerkx, A. H.E.M., Harchaoui, K. E., van der Steeg, W.A., et al. (2006) Cholesterol ester transfer protein (CETP) inhibition beyond raising high-density lipoprotein cholesterol levels. Arterioscler Thromb Vasc Biol. 26:706-715.

Kokkinos, P. F. (1999) Physical activity and high density lipoprotein cholesterol levels: what is the relationship? Sports Med. 28:307-314.

Lewis, G.F. and Rader, D.J. (2005) New insights into the regulation of HDL metabolism and reverse cholesterol transport. Circ. Res. 96:1221-1232.

Jerrod P. Libonati, MS, RD

Mackness, M.I., and Durrington, P.N. (1995) HDL, its enzymes and its potential to influence lipid peroxidation. Atherosclerosis. 115:243-253.

Muniyappa, R., Montagnani, M., Kon Koh, K., and Quon, M.J. (2007) Cardiovascular actions of insulin. Endocrine Reviews. 28:463-491.

Nathan, D.M., Davidson, M.B., DeFronzo, R.A. Heine, R.J., et al. (2007) Impaired fasting glucose and impaired glucose tolerance. Diabetes Care. 30:753-759.

Olofsson, S.O., Stillemark-Billton, P, and Asp, Lennart. (2000) Intracellular assembly of VLDL two major steps in separate compartments. Trends Cardiovasc Med. 10:338-345.

Rader, D.J. (2003) Regulation of reverse cholesterol transport and clinical implications. Am J Cardiol. 92(suppl):42J-49J.

Singh, I.M., Shishehbor, M.H., and Ansell, B.J. (2007) High density lipoprotein as a therapeutic target. JAMA. 298:786-798.

Unwin, N, Shaw, J., Zimmet, P., and Alberti, K.G.M.M. (2002) Impaired glucose tolerance and impaired fasting glycaemia: the current status on definition and intervention. Diabetes Medicine. 19:708-723.

Sherwin, R.S., Anderson, R.M., Buse, J.B. et al. (2002) The prevention or delay of type 2 diabetes. Diabetes Care. 4:742-749.

Sviridqv, D., and Nestle, P. (2002) Dynamics of reverse cholesterol transport: protection against atherosclerosis. Atherosclerosis. 161:245-254.

Tall, A.R. (1990) Plasma high density lipoproteins. J. Clin. Invest. 86:379-384.

Von Eckardstein, A., Nofer, J. R., and Assman, G. (2001) High density lipoproteins and arteriosclerosis: role of cholesterol efflux and reverse cholesterol transport. Arterioscler Thromb Vasc Biol. 21:13-27.

Windler, E., Schoffauer, M., and Zyriax, B.C. (2007) The significance of low HDL-cholesterol levels in an ageing society at increased risk for cardiovascular disease. Diabetes Vasc Dis Res. 4:136-142.

Yokoyama, S. (2006) Assembly of high-density lipoprotein. Arterioscler Thromb Vasc Biol. 26:20-27.

Section II   The Insulin Resistant State

Abdelmark, M.F., and Deihl, A.M. (2007) Nonalcoholic fatty liver disease as a complication of insulin resistance. Med Clin N Am 91:1125-1149.

Adeli, K., Taghibiglou, C, Van Iderstine, S.C., and Lewis, G.F. (2001) Mechanisms of hepatic very low-density lipoprotein overproduction in insulin resistance. Trends cardiovasc med. 11: 170-176.

Adler, A. I. (2002) Treating high blood pressure in diabetes: The evidence. Seminars in Vacular Medicine. 2 :127-137.

Babu, A., and Fogelfeld, L. (2006) Metabolic Syndrome and Prediabetes. Dis Mon. 52:55-114.

Barkis, G.L. (2007) Current perspectives on hypertension and metabolic syndrome. J Manag Care Pharm. 13:S3-S5.

Barter, P. (2006) Managing diabetic dyslipidemia-beyond LDL-C:HDL-C and triglycerides. Atheroscler Suppl. 7:17-21.

Basciano, H., Federico, L., and Adeli, K. (2005) Fructose, insulin resistance,and metabolic dyslipidemia. Nutrition & Metabolism. Feb 21; 2(1):5.

Baskin, M.L., Ard, J., Franklin, F., and Allison, D.B. (2005) Prevalence of obesity in the United States. Obes Rev. 6:5-7.

Bays, H. (2006) Clinical overview of omacor: a concentrated formulation of omega-3 polyunsaturated fatty acids. Am J Cardiol. 98 (Suppl.) 71i-76i.

Bernstein, A.M., Trezoyn, L., and Li, Z. (2007) Are high-protein, vegetable-based diets safe fro kidney function? A review of the literature. J Am Diet Assoc. 107:644-650.

Bock, G., Dalla Man, C., Campioni, M., Chittilapilly, E., et al. (2006) Mechanisms of fasting and postprandial hyperglycemia in people with impaired fasting glucose and/or impaired glucose tolerance. Diabetes. 55:3536-3549.

Boden, G., and Carnell, L.H. (2003) Nutritional effects of fat on carbohydrate metabolism. Best Pract & Res Clin Endocrinol Metab. 17:399-410.

Boden, G., and Shulman, G.I. (2002) Free fatty acids in obesity and type 2 diabetes: defining their role in the development of insulin resistance and beta-cell dysfunction. Eur J Clin Invest. 32 (Suppl.3) 14-23.

Borgman, M., and McErlean, E. (2006) What is the metabolic syndrome? Prediabetes and cardiovascular risk. J Cardio Nur. 21:285-290.

Castellani, L.W., Nguyen, C. N., Charugundla, S., Weinstein, M.W., et al. (2008) Apoliporotein A-II is a regulator of VLDL metabolism and insulin resistance. J Biol Chem. 283:11633-44.

Cersosimo, E., and DeFronzo, R.A. (2006) Insulin resistance and endothelial dysfunction: the road map to cardiovascular diseases. Diabetes Metab Res Rev. 22:423-436.

Chan, Juliana C.N., Tong, Peter C.Y., and Critchley, Julian A.J.H. (2002) The insulin resistance syndrome: Mechanisms of clustering of cardiovascular risk. 2:45-57.

Connelly, P.W. (1999) The role of hepatic lipase in lipoprotein metabolism. Clinica Chimica Acta. 286:243-255.

Corcoran, M.P., Fava-Lamon, Stefania., and Fielding, R.A. (2007) Skeletal muscle lipid deposition and insulin resistance: effect of dietary fatty acids and exercise. Am J Clin Nutr. 85: 662-77.

Davidson, M.H. (2006) Mechanisms for the hypotriglyceridemic effect of marine omega-3 fatty acids. Am J Cardiol. 98 (Suppl.1) 27i-33i.

DeFronzo, R. A. (2006) Is insulin resistance atherogenic? Possible mechanisms. Atherosclerosis Supplements. 7:11-15.

Desperes, J.P. (2006) Is visceral obesity the cause of the metabolic syndrome? Ann Med. 38:52-63.

Ferrannini, E., and Iozzo, P. (2006) Is insulin resistance atherogenic? A review of the evidence. Atherosclerosis Supplements. 7:5-10.

Fielding, C.J., and Fielding, P.E. (1995) Molecular physiology of reverse cholesterol transport. J. Lipid Res. 36:211-228.

Ford, E.S., Giles, W.H., and Dietz, W.H. (2002) Prevalence of the metabolic syndrome among US adults. Findings from the third national health and nutrition examination survey. JAMA. 287: 356-359.

Forrester, J.S., Makkar, R., and Shah, P.K. (2005) Increasing high-density lipoprotein cholesterol in dyslipidemia by cholesterol ester transfer protein inhibition. Circulation. 111:1847-1854.

Frayn, K.N. (2006) Visceral fat and insulin resistance-causative or correlative? Brit J Nutr. 83: (Suppl. 1) S71-77.

Frayn, K.N. (2005) Obesity and metabolic disease: is adipose tissue the culprit? Proceedings of the Nutr Soc. 64:7-13.

Ginsberg, H.N. (1996) Basic mechanisms underlying the common hypertriglyceridemia and low HDL cholesterol levels. Diabetes. 45 (Suppl. 3) S27-S30.

Ginsberg, H.N., Zhang, Y.L., and Hernandez-Ono, A. (2005) Regulation of plasma triglycerides in insulin resistance and diabetes. Archives of Med Res. 36:232-240.

Goodpaster, B.H., and Brown, N.F. (2005) Skeletal muscle lipid and its association with insulin resistance: what is the role for exercise? Exerc Sports Med Rev. 33:150-154.

Goossens, G.H. (2008) The role of adipose tissue dysfunction in the pathogenesis of obesity-related insulin resistance. Physiology & Behavior. 94:206-218.

Goldstein, B. (2003) Insulin resistance: from benign to type 2 diabetes mellitus. Rev Cardiovasc Med. 4: (Suppl. 6) S3-S10.

Greenberg, A.S., and McDaniel, M.L. (2002) Identifying the links between obesity, insulin resistance and beta cell function:potential role of adipocyte-derived cytokines in the pathogenesis of type 2 diabetes. Eur J Clin Invest. 32 (Suppl. 3) 24-34.

Groop, L., Forsblom, C., and Lehtovirta, M. (1997) Characterization of the prediabetic state. Am J Hypertens. 10:172s-180s.

Grundy, S.M., Cleeman, J.I., Daniels, S.R., Donato, K.A., et al. (2005) Diagnosis and management of the metabolic syndrome an American heart association/national heart, lung, and blood institute scientific statement. Cardiol Rev. Nov-Dec. 13:322-327.

Haffner, S.M. (2003) Pre-diabetes, insulin resistance, inflammation and CVD risk. Diab Res Clin Pract. 61:S9-S18.

Haffner, S.M. (1999) Epidemiology of insulin resistance and its relation to coronary artery disease. Am J Cardiol. 84:11J-14J.

Haffner, S., and Taegtmeyer, H. (2003) Epidemic obesity and the metabolic syndrome. Circulation. 108:1541-1545.

Havel, P.J. (2000) Role of adipose tissue in body-weight regulation: mechanisms regulating leptin production and energy balance. Proc Nutr Soc. 59:359-371.

Hollander, J.M., and Mechanick, J.I. (2008) Complimentary and alternative medicine and the management of the metabolic syndrome. J Am Diet Assoc. 108:495-509.

Hseuh, W. A., Lyon, C.J., and Quinones, M.J. (2004) Insulin resistance and the endothelium. Am J Med. 117:109-117.

Hsueh, W.A., and Quinones, M.J. (2003) Role of endothelial dysfunction in insulin resistance. Am J Cardiol. 92: (Suppl.) 10J-17J.

Jansson, P.A. (2007) Endothelial dysfunction in insulin resistance and type 2 diabetes. J Intern Med. 262: 173-183.

Jequier, E., and Tappy, L. (1999) Regulation of body weight in humans. Physiol Rev. 79:451-480.

Jeukendrop, A.E. (2002) Regulation of fat metabolism in skeletal muscle. Ann NY. Sci. 967:217-235.

Keller, U. (2006) From Obesity to Diabetes. Int. J. Vitam. Nutr. Res. 76:172-177.

Kelly. D.E., Goodpaster, B.H., and Storlien, L. (2002) Muscle triglyceride and insulin resistance. Annu Rev Nutr. 22:325-46.

Kereiakes, D.J. and Willerson, J.T. (2003) Metabolic syndrome epidemic. Circulation. 108:1552-1553.

Kiens, B., and Lithell, H. (1989) Lipoprotein metabolism influenced by training-induced changes in human skeletal muscle. J Clin Invest. 83:558-564.

Kim, J. A., Montagnami, M., Koh, K.K. and Quon, M.J. (2006) Reciprocal relationships between insulin resistance and endothelial dysfunction. Molecular and pathophysiological mechanisms. Circulation. 113:1888-1904.

Kraegen, E.W., Cooney, G.J., Ye, J., and Thompson, A.L. (2001) Triglycerides, fatty acids and insulin resistance-hyperinsulinemia. Exp Clin Endocrinol Diabetes. 109:S516-S526.

Krause, B.R., and Hartman, A.D. (1984) Adipose tissue and cholesterol metabolism. J. Lipid Res. 25:97-110.

Kraus, W.E., Houmard, J.A., Duscha, B.D., Knetzger, K.J., et al. (2002) Effects of the amount and intensity of exercise on plasma lipoproteins. N Eng J Med. 347:1483-92.

Lamarche, B., and Paradis, M.E. (2007) Endothelial lipase and the metabolic syndrome. Curr Opin Lipidol. 18:298-303.

Lamarche, B., Rashid, S,. and Lewis, G.F. (1999) HDL metabolism in hypertriglyceridemc states:an overview. Clinica Chimica Acta. 286:145-161.

Lehman, R., Engler, H., Honegger, R., Riesen, W., et al. (2001) Alterations of lipolytic enzymes and high-density lipoprotein subfractions induced by physical activity in type 2 diabetes. Eur J Clin Invest. 31:37-44.

Lewis, G.F., Carpentier, A., Adeli, K., and Giacca, A. (2002) Disordered fat storage and mobilization in the pathogenesis of insulin resistance and type 2 diabetes. Endo Rev. 23: 201-229.

Lewis, G.F. and Steiner, G. (1996) Hypertriglyceridemia and its metabolic consequences as a risk facto for atherosclerotic cardiovascular disease in non-insulin dependent diabetes mellitus. Diabetes Met Rev. 12:37-56.

Liberopoulous, E.N., Mikhailidis, D.P., and Elisaf, M.S. (2005) Diagnosis and management of the metabolic syndrome in obesity. Obesity Rev. 6:283-296.

Link, J.J., Rohatgi, A., and de Lemos, J.A. (2007) HDL cholesterol: physiology, pathophysiology, and management. Curr Probl Cardiol. 32:268-314.

Madamanchi, N.R., and Runge, M.S. (2006) Five Easy Pieces The obesity paradigm. Circ Res. 98:576-578.

McCarty, M.F. (2003) A paradox resolved: the postprandial model of insulin resistance explains why gynoid adiposity appears to be protective. Med Hypotheses. 61:173-176.

McKenney, J.A., and Sica, D. (2007) Prescription omega-3 fatty acids for the treatment of hypertriglyceridemia. Am J Health-Syst Pharm. 64:595-605.

Moore, M.C. (2003) Regulation of hepatic and peripheral glucose disposal. Best Pract Res Clin Endocrin Metab. 17:343-364.

Olchawa, B., Kingwell, B.A., Hoang, A., Schneider, L., et al. (2004) Physical fitness and reverse cholesterol transport. Arterioscler Thromb Vasc Biol. 24: 1087-1091.

Paglialunga, S., and Cianflone, K. (2007) Regulation of postprandial lipemia: an update on current trends. Appl Physiol Nutr Metab. 32:61-75.

Qureshi, K., and Abrams, G.A. (2007) Metabolic liver disease of obesity and role of adipose tissue in the pathogenesis of nonalcoholic fatty liver disease. World J Gastroenterol. 13:3540-3553.

Rashid, S., Watanabe, T., Sakaue, T., and Lewis, G.F. (2003) Mechanisms of HDL lowering in insulin resistant, hypertriglyceridemic states: the combined effect of HDL triglyceride enrichment and elevated hepatic lipase activity. Clin Biochem. 36:421-429.

Rashid, S., Uffelman, K.D., and Lewis, G.F. (2002) The mechanism of HDL lowering in hypertriglyceridemic, insulin resistant states. J Diabetes Compl. 16:24-28.

Ravussin, E., and Smith, S.R. (2002) Increased fat intake, impaired fat oxidation, and failure of fat cell proliferation result in ectopic fat storage, insulin resistance, and type 2 diabetes mellitus. Ann NY Acad Sci. 967:363-378.

Roden, M., and Bernroider, E. (2003) Hepatic glucose metabolism in humans-its role in health and disease. Best Pract Res Clin Endocrin Metab. 17:365-383.

Roche, H. M. (2005) Fatty acids and the metabolic syndrome. Proceedings of the Nutr Soc. 64: 23-29.

Raz, I., Eldor, R., Cernea, S., and Shafrir, E. (2005) Diabetes: insulin resistance and derangements in lipid metabolism. Cure through intervention in fat transport and storage. Diabetes Met Rev. 21:3-14.

Reaven, G.M. (1995) Pathophysiology of insulin resistance in human disease. Physiol Rev. 75: 473-486.

Reaven, G.M. (1988) Role of insulin resistance in human disease. Diabetes. 37:1595-1607.

Robinson, L.E., Buchholz, A.C., and Mazurak, V.C. (2007) Inflammation, obesity, and fatty acid metabolism: influence of n-3 polyunsaturated fatty acids on factors contributing to metabolic syndrome. Appl Physiol Nutr Metab. 32:1008-1024.

Sahib, A.K., Sahu, S., and Reddy, K.N. (2007) Prediabetes and hypertension. J Indian Med Assoc. 105:25-28.

Saleh, J., Sniderman, A.D., and Cianflone, K. (1999) Regulation of plasma fatty acid metabolism. Clinica Chimica Acta. 286:163-180.

Saloranta, C., and Groop, L. (1996) Interactions between glucose and ffa metabolism in man. Diabetes Met Rev. 12:15-36.

Sato, Y. (2000) Diabetes and life-styles: role of physical exercise for primary prevention. Br J Nutr. 84: (Suppl. 2) S187-190.

Stannard, S.R., and Johnson, N.A. (2003) Insulin resistance and elevated triglycerides in muscle: more important for survival than "thrifty" genes? J Physiol. 554:595-607.

Tall, A.R. (2002) Exercise to reduce cardiovascular risk-how much is enough? N Engl J Med. 347:1522- 1524.

Tall, A.R. (1993) Plasma cholesterol ester transfer protein. J Lipid Res. 34: 1255-1274.

Taskinen, M.R. (2003) LDL-cholesterol, HDL-cholesterol or triglycerides-which is the culprit. Diabetes Res Clin Pract. 61:S19-S26.

Tierney, A.C., and Roche, H.M. (2007) The potential role of olive oil-derived MUFA in insulin sensitivity. Mol Nutr Food Res. 51:1235-1248.

Trayhurn, P. (2005) Endocrine and signaling role of adipose tissue:new perspectives on fat. Acta Physiol Scand. 184:285-293.

Vita, J.A. (2000) Exercise-toning up the endothelium? N Eng J Med. 342:503-505.

Williams, C.M., Maitin, V., and Jackson, K.G. (2004) Triacylglycerol-rich lipoprotein-gene interactions in endothelial cells. Biochem Soc Trans. 32:994-998.

Wilson, P.W.F., and Grundy, S.M. (2003) The metabolic syndrome a practical guide to origins and treatment: part I. Circulation. 108:1422-1425.

Wilson, P.W.F., and Grundy, S.M. (2003) The metabolic syndrome a practical guide to origins and treatment: part II. Circulation. 108:1537-1540.

Wing, R. R., and Phelan, S. (2005) Long-term weight loss maintenance. Am J Clin Nutr. 82: (Suppl.) 222S-225S.

Wedick, N.M., Mayer-Davis, E., Winguard, D.L. Addy, C.L., et al. (2001) Insulin resistance precedes weight loss in adults without diabetes. Am J Epidemiol. 153:1199-1205.

Weiss, R. (2007) Fat distribution and storage: how much, where, and how? Eur J Endocrinol 157: S39-S45.

Weyer, C., Hanson, K., Bogardus, C., and Pratley, R.E. (2000) Long-term changes in insulin action and insulin secretion associated with gain, loss, regain and maintenance of body weight. Diabetologia. 43:36-46.

Wheatcroft, S.B., Williams, I. L., Shah, A.M., and Kearney, M.T. (2003) Pahtophysiological implications of insulin resistance on vascular endothelial function. Diabet Med. 20:255-268.

Ye, J., and Kreagen, T. (2008) Insulin resistance: central and peripheral mechanisms. The 2007 stock conference report. Obes Rev. 9:30-34.

Yuan, G., Al-Shali, K. Z., and Hegele, R.A. (2007) Hypertriglyceridemia: its etiology, effects and treatment. CMAJ. 176:1113-20.

Zierath, J.R., and Kawano, Y. (2003) The effect of hyperglycemia on glucose disposal and insulin signal transduction in skeletal muscle. Best Pract Res Clin Endocrin Metab. 17:385-398.

Section III   The Diet Controversy

Bantle, J.P., Wylie-Rosett, J., Albright, A.L., Apovian, C.M., et al. (2007) Nutrition recommendations and interventions for diabetes. Diabetes Care. 30: (Suppl.1) S48-S65.

Brunner, E.J., Wunsch, H., and Marmot, M.G. (2001) What is the optimal diet? Relationship of macronutrient intake to obesity, glucose tolerance, lipoprotein cholesterol levels and the metabolic syndrome in the Whitehall II study. Int J Obes. 25:45-53.

Calder, P.C., and Deckelbaum, R.J. (2008) Omega-3 fatty acids: time to get the message right! Curr Opin Clin Nutr Metab Care. 11:91-93.

Dansinger, M.L., Gleason, J. L., Griffith, J.L., Selker, H.P., and Schaefer, E.J. (2005) Comparison of the atkins, ornish, weight watchers, and zone diets for weight loss and heart disease risk reduction. JAMA. 293:43-53.

Donovan, D.S., Solomon, C.G., Seely, E.W., Williams, G.H., and Simonson, D.C. (1993) Effect of sodium intake on insulin sensitivity. Endocrinol Metab. 264:E730-E734.

Esmaillzadeh, A., Kimiagar, M., Mehrabi, Y., Azadbakht, L., et al. (2006) Fruit and vegetable intakes, c-reactive protein, and the metabolic syndrome. Am J Clin Nutr. 84:1489-97.

Esposito, K., Ciotola, M., and Giugliano, D. (2007) Mediterranean diet and the metabolic syndrome. Mol Nutr Res. 51:1268-1274.

Feldeisen, S.E., and Tucker, K.L. (2007) Nutritional strategies in the prevention and treatment of the metabolic syndrome. 32:46-60.

Foster-Powell, K., Holt, S.H.A., and Brand-Miller, J.C. (2002) International table of glycemic index and glycemic load values: 2002. 76:5-56.

Franz, M.J. (2003) So many nutrition recommendations-contradictory or compatible? Diabetes Spectrum. 16:56-63.

Franz, M.J., Bantle, J.P., Beebe, C. A., Brunzell, J.D., et al. (2002) Evidence-based nutrition principles and recommendations for the treatment and prevention of diabetes and related complications. Diabetes Care. 25 (Suppl. 1) S50-S60.

Frost, G., Leeds, A.A., Dore, C.J., Madeiros, S., et al. (1999) Glycaemic index as a determinant of serum HDL-cholesterol concentration. Lancet. 353:1045-48.

Griel, A.E., Ruder, E.H., and Kris-Etherton, P.M. (2006) The changing role of dietary carbohydrates from simple to complex. Arterioscler Thromb Vasc Biol. 26:1958-1965.

Hagura, R. (2000) Diabetes mellitus and life-style-for the primary prevention of diabetes mellitus: the role of diet. 84 (Suppl.) S191-S194.

Hallikainen, M., Toppinen, L., Mykkanen, H., Agren, J.J., et al. (2006) Interaction between cholesterol and glucose metabolism during dietary carbohydrate modification in subjects with the metabolic syndrome. 84:1385-92.

Kennedy, E.T., Bowman, S., Spence, J.T., Freedman, M., et al. (2001) Popular diets: correlation to health, nutrition and obesity. J Am Diet Assoc. 101:411-420.

Kirk, J.K., Graves, D.E., Craven, T.E., Lipkin, E.W., et al. (2008) Restricted-carbohydrate diets in patients with type 2 diabetes: a meta analysis. J Am Diet Assoc. 108:91-100.

Kopp, W. (2006) The atherogenic potential role of dietary carbohydrate. Prev Med. 42:336-342.

Lara-Castro, C., and Garvey, T. (2004) Diet, insulin resistance and obesity: zoning in on data for atkins dieters living in south beach. J Clin Endocrinol Metab. 89:4197-4205.

Lee, J.S., Pinnamaneni, S.J.E., Cho, I.H., Pyo, J.H., et al. (2006) Saturated, but not n-6 polyunsaturated, fatty acids induce insulin resistance: role of intramuscular accumulation of lipid metabolites. J Appl Physiol. 100:1467-1474.

Lichtenstein, A.H. (2006) Dietary fat, carbohydrate, and protein: effects on plasma lipoprotein patterns. J Lipid Res. 47:1661-1667.

Liese, A.D., Gilliard, T., Schulz, M., D'Agostino, R.B., et al, (2007) Carbohydrate nutrition, glycemic load, and plasma lipids: the insulin resistance atherosclerosis study. Eur Heart Journal. 28:80-87.

Ludwig, D.S. (2002) The glycemic index. JAMA. 287:2414-2423.

Marshall, J.A., Bessesen, D.H., and Hamman, R.F. (1997) High saturated fat and low starch and fibre are associated with hyperinsulinemia in a non-diabetic population: the san luis valley diabetes study. Diabetologia. 40:430-438.

Martini, L.A., and Wood, R.J. (2006) Vitamin D status and the metabolic syndrome. Nutr Reviews. 64:479-486.

McAuley, K., and Mann, J. (2006) Nutritional determinants of insulin resistance. J Lipid Res. 47: 1668-1676.

Mobbs, C.V., Mastaitis, J., Schwartz, J., Mohan, V., et al. (2007) Low-carbohydrate diets cause obesity, low-carbohydrate diets reverse obesity: A metabolic mechanism resolving the paradox. Appetite. 48:135-138.

Nordmann, A.J., Nordman, A., Briel, M., Keller, U., et al. (2006) Effects of low-carbohydrate vs low-fat diets on weight loss and cardiovascular risk factors. Arch Intern Med. 166:285-293.

Ohlson, M.S. (2006) The skinny on low-carbohydrate diets. J Cardiovasc Nurs. 21:314-321.

Panagiotakos, D.B., Pitsavos, C., Skoumas, Y., and Stefanadis, C. (2007) The association between food patterns and the metabolic syndrome using principal components analysis: the attica study. J Am Diet Assoc. 107:979-987.

Pfeuffer, M., and Schrezenmeir, J. (2006) Milk and the metabolic syndrome. Obes Rev. 8:109-118.

Pittas, A.G., and Roberts, S.B. (2006) Dietary composition and weight loss: can we individualize dietary prescriptions according to insulin sensitivity or secretion status? Nutr Rev. 64:435-448.

Qi, L., and Hu, F.B. (2007) Dietary glycemic load, whole grains, and systemic inflammation in diabetes: the epidemiological evidence. Curr Opin Lipidol. 18:3-8.

Riccardi, G., and Rivellese, A.A. (2000) Dietary treatment of the metabolic syndrome-the optimal diet. Br J Nutr. 83 (Suppl.1) S143-S148.

Rivellese, A.A., De Natale, C., and Lilli, S. (2002) Type of dietary fat and insulin resistance. Ann NY Acad Sci. 967:329-335.

Selmi, C., Bowlus, C.L., Keen, C.L. and Gershwin, M.E. (2007) Non-alchoholic fatty liver disease: the new epidemic and the need for novel nutritional approaches. J Med Food. 10:563-565.

Swain, J.F., McCarron, P.B., Hamilton, E.F., Sacks, F.M., et al. (2008) Characteristics of the diet patterns tested in the optimal macronutrient intake trial to prevent heart disease (omniheart): options for a heart healthy diet. J Am Diet Assoc. 108:257-265.

Van Horn, L., McCoin, M., Kris-Etherton, P.M., Burke, F., et al. (2008) The evidence for dietary prevention and treatment of cardiovascular disease. J Am Diet Assoc. 108: 287-331.

Wood, R.J. (2006) Effect of dietary carbohydrate restriction with and without weight loss on atherogenic dyslipidemia. Nutr Rev. 64:539-545.

Wood, R.J., Volek, J.S., Liu, Y., Shachter, N.S., et al. (2006) Carbohydrate restriction alters lipoprotein metabolism by modifying VLDL, LDL and HDL subfraction distribution and size in overweight men. J Nutr. 136:384-389.

www.ingramcontent.com/pod-product-compliance
Lightning Source LLC
Chambersburg PA
CBHW032005170526
45157CB00002B/561